Working Whole Systems

Putting theory into practice in organisations

Related titles:

Working Whole Systems

Putting theory into practice in organisations

Julian Pratt, Pat Gordon and Diane Plamping

Foreword by Margaret J. Wheatley

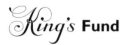

King's Fund

Published by
King's Fund Publishing
11–13 Cavendish Square
London W1M 0AN

© King's Fund 1999

First published 1999

ISBN 1 85717 233 7

A CIP catalogue record for this book is available from the British Library

Available from:

King's Fund Bookshop
11–13 Cavendish Square
London
W1M 0AN

Tel: 0171 307 2591
Fax: 0171 307 2801

Printed and bound in Great Britain

Cover illustration: Creativ Collection
Text photographs: King's Fund, John Birdsall, Joanne O'Brien/Format,
Karen Robinson/Format

Contents

Events

Where to begin?

Where we began

Foreword

I was delighted to read this book. It is simply the most thoughtful, comprehensible, and accessible work I have yet seen on working with the whole system. Its authors speak from their hard-won wisdom; as you read their comments, you know you are in the presence of people who have been doing the work for a long time and spent long hours reflecting on its meaning and lessons.

The field of whole systems work offers great hope, because it demonstrates that when the entire organisation or community is engaged in the work of planning its own future, wondrous possibilities emerge. This is no exaggeration; people who engage the whole of a system always use the word 'miraculous' to describe the results of the experience. And we really need new models for coming together. Everyone has grown tired of endless meetings, recurring conflicts, bad behaviours, heroic leaders and problems that get larger rather than resolved. We cannot move into any future worth wanting with our old group processes; we need to learn more about how to bring people together in the systems of relationships that give birth to new possibilities.

This is the era of fractured relationships: leaders don't trust their workers; we don't trust each other; intractable problems refuse to be solved by piecemeal approaches. Our work is truly to reweave the world – to call together those who have kept apart, to understand problems in all their rich dimensions, to become sensitive to how systems move and change. In this work, we are only recalling ourselves to an old memory, the remembrance of working together for the common community and developing systems of relationships that sustain us individually and collectively. We are only remembering how Life organises, and experimenting with how to bring that wisdom back into our organisational processes.

In reading this book, you will not only learn particular processes for bringing the whole of a system together; you will also learn a great deal about how living systems grow and change. The work described in these pages is grounded in an emerging theory of living systems and the organising processes that lead to capacity, resiliency and adaptability. It is refreshing to read a book that goes beyond simple lists and 'how-tos' and grounds its assertions in a deeper theory. In this way, the authors ask us to engage with them in a serious and ongoing inquiry into new ways of organising. They invite each of us to contribute our curiosity, our intelligence and our desire to find new ways of working together. It is an important invitation and one that I hope you as readers accept.

Margaret J Wheatley

Acknowledgements

Many, many people have contributed to the work and the ideas on which this book is based – some as members of the core development group, others in local sites, on steering groups, funding bodies, workshop programmes, evaluation teams and as wise advisers and commentators. Some have patiently read and re-read early drafts of the book and others have creatively edited and designed it. Our thanks are due to all of them and in particular to Giovanna Ceroni, Elsie Cliff, Barbara Douglas, Kathryn Evans, Angela Everitt, Martin Fischer, John Harries, Maggie Jee, Myron Kellner-Rogers, Iain Kitt, Sue Lloyd-Evelyn, Minuche Mazumdar Farrar, Dave Martin, Jane Neubauer, Sharon Ombler-Spain, Jennie Popay, Peter Reason, Jenny Rogers, Madeleine Rooke-Ley and Meg Wheatley.

Above all, we want to thank the many courageous people in local agencies who were looking for new ways of working and recognised that nothing much would change if 'we go on doing more of the same'. They took the risk of embarking on this venture with us when all we had to offer were ideas, a modest amount of grant money and a fair degree of hassle. Without them there would be nothing to say.

Julian Pratt
Diane Plamping
Pat Gordon

Introduction and how to use this book

This book offers a radical way of thinking about organisations as living systems, and practical methods of engaging with complex social and organisational issues. We call the approach we have developed *Working Whole Systems*. It is based on four years' experience of learning how to put theory into practice in Liverpool, London and Newcastle and North Tyneside.

Working Whole Systems is likely to interest you if you are looking for new ways of working. We imagine you, the reader, as a sceptical optimist. Your concerns may be about productive partnerships or genuinely engaging local people or involving far more people than usual in building strategy or creating energy for sustainable change. You know there aren't any 'quick fixes'. You recognise that 'more of the same' is not going to be enough and you are curious about why some problems keep returning to haunt us despite the hard work and good intentions of many people. We hope you find ideas in this book which rekindle your enthusiasms, as they have ours.

Our work has been with health agencies and their local partners in housing, transport, local government, the independent sector, the police, voluntary agencies, and local citizens. The whole system approach we have developed always involves working with many types of stakeholder. It always engages local people in active participation and it sometimes includes working with large numbers of people simultaneously. Its purpose is to find local solutions to local concerns.

The development programme which generated the work is described on page 153. Its focus was improving services for older people in three cities in the UK and many of the examples in the book are drawn from this experience. However, the concepts and the practical working methods we describe are widely applicable wherever people are searching for new ways of working on seemingly intractable issues.

How to use this book ...

We imagine readers will have varying degrees of first-hand experience of working from a whole system perspective, and so the book is written to be read in different ways. You may find it most satisfactory to read the chapters in sequence, but they can be taken in any order.

If you want a flavour of this way of working, turn to the *Story* on page 79. If your particular interest is designs for large group meetings you may want to begin with the chapter on *Events*. If the underlying theory interests you, you may choose to start with *Metaphors*. If you are not sure whether this is something you even want to consider, then we suggest you start with the first, short chapter on *Working Whole Systems* where we try to distil what we mean by the whole system approach. You will know by the end of these three pages whether this book is for you.

For us the book is work-in-progress. We try to develop our understanding of both theory and action by repeatedly trying them out against each other and the book describes where we have got to towards the end of 1998. It is also an open invitation to contact us at: wws@dial.pipex.com if you are interested in engaging further with the ideas you find here.

Glossary

In this book we use some everyday words in quite particular ways:

Communication   an activity that co-ordinates a change in behaviour. This is not simply the transmission of information

Complex   describes something that is more than just 'complicated'. Both words have a shared derivation, but 'complex' is also derived from the Latin verb complectere (to encompass, embrace, enclose, comprehend, comprise). It has a sense of a whole, of various parts connected together, as is suggested by the use of the term 'building complex'. When a complex whole is analysed into parts the parts themselves are complex not simple – organisations are made up of groups, groups made up of people, people made up of cells, cells made up of organelles, organelles made up of complex catalytic systems ... It is not possible to predict the detailed behaviour of a complex whole from an understanding of these parts, though it is possible to anticipate patterns of order.

Complicated   we use 'complicated' as the antonym of 'simple'. It is derived from com (with) + plicare (to fold) and so has the sense of 'folded, wrapped or twisted together, mixed up in an involved way'. We might describe the street map of a city centre or the inside of a TV set as 'complicated' to mean how it is 'mixed up in an involved way'. Something that is complicated can, at least in principle, be analysed into parts that are simple. No matter how many parts and how many connections there are, it is possible, in principle, to predict the behaviour of the whole.

Dialogue	dialogue is a conversation in which a group 'thinks together', allowing itself to discover insights that might not be accessible to its members thinking individually. We use it by contrast with 'discussion', the process of examining the arguments for and against some proposition. Dialogue is also a specific approach to communication which recognises patterns of interaction that inhibit learning, makes explicit people's internal assumptions and works with these.
Human system	a system containing people
Lay people	people who contribute from their experience of living their lives in this or that place – it includes citizens and people who use services. In this book we use it interchangeably with 'elders' or 'older people' as the particular programme of work we describe focused on this group of lay people.
Learning organisation	an organisation that is continually expanding its capacity to create its future. This depends on the behaviour of the organisation, not just how much information it has.
Mental map/mental model	the set of assumptions, beliefs, images and stories that influence how a person understands the world and how they take action.
Organisation	we use this word in two different ways. Usually we use it in its everyday sense of a business, institution or agency. We sometimes refer to 'organisation' in the sense that it is used by Maturana, as the 'configuration of relationships among the system's components that determine the system's essential characteristics'. When we use the word in this way we follow Capra and use the phrase 'pattern of organisation'.

Professionals   people who contribute from their experience of working to provide services or goods for others (whether paid or unpaid). It includes people who might describe themselves as managers or receptionists, clinicians or volunteers. It includes people working in the statutory, voluntary and commercial sectors.

System   we use this word in two different ways. Usually, we refer to a human system of a particular type. Here we use it to mean something that assembles itself around shared meaning and purpose, such as the quality of life for older people in a neighbourhood. We do not use the word 'system' in the sense of a fixed organisational structure such as a telephone system, a benefits system or a hospital. We also use the word in its most general sense as 'a perceived whole whose essential properties arise from the relationships between its parts'.

Working Whole Systems

WHOLE SYSTEM WORKING IS A RADICAL WAY OF THINKING ABOUT
CHANGE IN COMPLEX SITUATIONS; A COMBINATION OF THEORY
AND PRACTICAL METHODS OF WORKING ACROSS BOUNDARIES

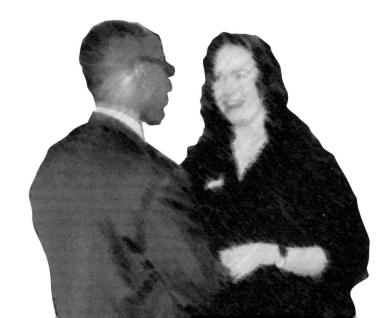

'Whole system working' helps people make organisational connections that enable them to find sustainable local solutions to local concerns. These connections are with both people and ideas.

At its simplest level, whole system working is a way of thinking about and designing meetings that help people to express their different experiences, to identify possibilities for action and to commit to change. At a more profound level, it is an approach to organisational development that views groups of people who come together around a shared purpose as living systems. It recognises that the way in which living systems adapt and evolve is determined by the way interconnected parts relate to each other, as well as the way individual parts behave.

Whole system working shifts the focus of attention from parts to 'the whole' and offers a set of practical working methods to influence the way 'the parts' connect and behave towards each other.

From the parts to the whole

Complex social issues such as urban regeneration, homelessness, underachievement in schools or long-term unemployment are influenced by the actions of many individuals, groups and organisations. They are beyond the ability of any one agency or individual 'to fix'. In trying to tackle them the tendency is to break them into actionable parts. Yet despite the hard work of policy-makers and good people 'on the ground', many of these problems refuse to go away. They keep coming round again and again. We reasoned that it might be more fruitful to think of them as issues for an interconnected system to tackle together. We chose to shift our attention from parts on to the whole and thus to the connections between parts – how things fit together. This awareness means having to have a picture or model of what systems are like.

Organisations as living systems

Metaphors provide useful ways of thinking about organisations and how they work. We have used metaphors derived from living systems like organisms, ecosystems and brains. This leads us to think of individuals, teams, departments and organisations as purposeful entities linked in a web of interdependence. We think they can interact intelligently, autonomously and through a process of constantly adapting to each other. They are not limited to behaving in ways predetermined by a designer, planner or chief executive.

In drawing on our understanding of living systems we are interested in 'how things get done'. We assume that change is ever present and that people tend naturally towards change and development. We do not believe that change is always resisted and therefore has to 'be managed'. We are seeking very practical answers to some of the questions raised in the growing body of literature on 'the new science' and its applicability to organisational and social life. In their book, *A Simpler Way*, for example, Margaret Wheatley and Myron Kellner-Rogers elegantly address the question: 'How could we organise human endeavour if we developed different understandings of how life organises itself?'

Meetings for different purposes

People and organisations get much of their work done in face-to-face meetings. Of course there are other ways of operating and people may undertake much day-to-day activity on their own or with clients. But it is in meetings that people share, discuss, connect, relate and make decisions – with or without the support of facts and figures, budgets and papers.

And yet ... so often meetings are seen as time-wasting and frustrating. Do there have to be so many? What is it we *really* need to meet about? Could we organise them differently? Could we do business another way? By drawing on our understanding of living systems we have explored ways of thinking about and designing meetings that are different from those traditionally used for formal decision-making.

Whole system meetings may be large or small. They are designed to enable people to recognise shared purpose in what they do, and to make connections and explore possibilities for action. Sometimes large numbers of people assemble to work together and we call these occasions 'whole system events'. These are not isolated events but highly visible moments in a much longer process. They enable lots of people to become aware of being part of a wider system.

In summary ... In this chapter we have tried to distil what we mean by whole system working. It is an approach to the way people organise their work together. It is a combination of theory and practical methods for working across boundaries. It is a way of seeing the world from which certain actions flow. It can be a means of enabling local people to find solutions to local concerns without the need for injections of external knowledge and resources.

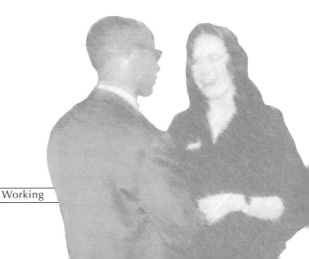

Metaphors

IF YOU THINK OF ORGANISATIONS AS LIVING SYSTEMS,
YOU PAY ATTENTION TO CERTAIN
FEATURES SUCH AS CONNECTIONS,
RELATIONSHIPS, MEANING.
IF YOU THINK OF MECHANICAL SYSTEMS,
YOU PAY ATTENTION TO DESIGN,
CONTROL MECHANISMS AND SO ON

Our beliefs about the way the world works influence what we do and what we can imagine doing. They open up or close down possible courses of action, which 'depend on how you see things'. Metaphor is a way of illuminating our thinking about the world, and in this chapter we look at two useful and contrasting metaphors for the way organisations work, and therefore the ways in which we might act if we wanted to change their behaviour.

We have become used to the language of mechanical systems when we talk of organisational behaviour – cogs and wheels, oil, transmission, levers, re-design and so on. The hierarchical structure of many organisations reflects this (Fig. 1). At the top of a pyramid are the designers: the CEO and board, responsible for identifying the goals of the organisation and the ways of achieving them. At the bottom are the operational workers, responsible for 'playing their part'. Between these levels are managers, oiling the wheels – transmitting information up and down, identifying problems, proposing and then implementing solutions, and monitoring the outcomes.

Fig. 1 **Hierarchical structure**

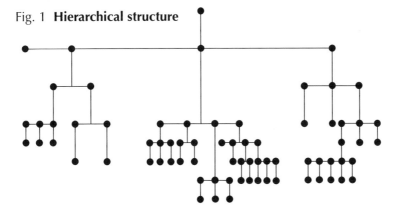

This management practice is based on scientific ideas which have increased our understanding of the world by their ability to break activities into their component parts. These parts can then be standardised and optimised and re-assembled. Organisations generally use serial or sequential processes. Optimising such a system and increasing its efficiency consist of improving the speed and quality of each stage.

When you think of an organisation as a mechanical system, you think of change as an 'effect' that arises in a way that can be traced back to a 'cause'. The appropriate system behaviour is sequential – analysis, planning, action and review that occur one after the other, feeding into further cycles. The people best placed to control these activities are at the top of the organisation.

Machines

A machine has a designer who specifies the parts and how these interact. Only the designer needs to know how the whole works. The machine needs engineers to maintain it. And if it is to be used for a new purpose it has to be redesigned and re-engineered. The reason is that machines do not organise and maintain themselves, they do not naturally adapt to changing environments. Indeed, left to themselves, machines tend to deteriorate and their performance declines.

The parts of the machine are generally responsive rather than initiating action. They are expected to 'play their part', no more and no less. The machine works predominantly in sequence. It works as a whole because the relationships between the parts is designed in.

Information flows between the parts of the whole. The science of information theory has improved our understanding of the transmission of information, emphasising the importance of the quality of the data transmitted, its appropriateness to the receiver, and the clarity of the transmission channel.

Within the organisation there are inevitably many different perspectives. One way to bring these together is to find an outside expert to build up a rich understanding of the way the whole system works that will be useful to all those involved. The expert might gather information from different sorts of people, by using surveys and questionnaires as well as interviews. And they might build up a word-picture, a report, a computer model to summarise and feed back what they have learned. There are many ways of carrying out this sequence of research and development.

This approach becomes increasingly problematic as the system becomes more complex and the number of perspectives or mental maps that the expert has to fit together into a master-map increases. There are several reasons for this:

- different maps may be appropriately used for different purposes and there may even be no need to produce a single map
- while there is much to be gained from a simple model of a complex whole, there is a risk that it may be simplistic and fail to capture the complexity. Insights based on a simplistic model may lead to unexpected consequences for other parts of the system and for the system as a whole
- the 'expert' approach may take a long time, and the system may have changed radically before the expert reports back
- it is the expert who learns about the system, not those who play their part in it. Research may influence practice, but there is no necessary linkage between the expert's analysis and the system's capacity to change.

When organisations are designed using the machine as the dominant metaphor, those at the top of the hierarchy have power and change is a top-down process. If the organisation assumes that operational workers simply respond rather than move things forward themselves, key management roles are monitoring, control and 'motivation'. Co-ordination between different organisations requires joint strategy, joint planning and sometimes joint funding.

The course of change is punctuated by meetings, but most of the 'real' work is done between meetings. One person (or department or organisation) prepares a draft which is circulated for consultation and refined. Good meetings rely on good preparation and provide a mechanism for tidying up – for legitimising (or challenging) the next steps, which occur outside the meeting.

Interaction takes place between levels of a hierarchy but often on terms set by the powerful. Feedback, for example, is a mechanism whereby line managers listen to the experiences of those they are managing and relay these upwards. Consultation can be a means of discovering the opinions of lay people in order to improve services. Organisations may even encourage bottom-up community development activities to complement their top-down approach. The organisation may also consult with citizens in order to gain democratic legitimacy. This requires that the consulted are representative of the whole group.

Formal control mechanisms frequently generate opposition. Recognising that power lies at the top of the organisation, people respond by trying to exert influence at this level. This generally takes the form of campaigning, challenge, and 'holding the leaders to account'. There are alliances, but they are often 'alliances against', not 'alliances for'. Hierarchical structures are effective ways of getting some things done but they have important limitations:

- they are well designed to control but less good at adapting

- they may be effective in ensuring compliance, but they are not good at encouraging creativity

- the legitimacy of power may be uncontested in a single organisational structure, but this is unlikely to be the case in partnerships involving other organisations

- because it is difficult to consult with *all* the people who live in an area or work in an organisation, consultation frequently takes place with representatives who speak for the others. These may be campaigning groups and voluntary organisations who derive their legitimacy from their claim to speak *for* a group of citizens or trade unions to speak *for* their members.

The machine metaphor is not so well suited to complex situations in which any change may give rise to unintended consequences. If 'the whole' cannot be understood through a better understanding of the component parts, then a new approach is needed, and this is now well understood. In the complex world we really live in 'things bite back', as Edward Tenner demonstrates in his book *Why Things Bite Back: New technology and the revenge effect*.

Living systems

We all have direct experience of whole organisms like animals and plants and some awareness of the nature of other living systems like cells and ecosystems. An unambiguous definition of life may not be easy but broadly speaking we can recognise its characteristics, which are described more formally in the appendix to this chapter.

Living systems are generally 'on the move' – growing, moving, repairing, changing, adapting, reproducing, evolving. They are 'hungry', they need to be able to take in energy and use it to keep going. We may intervene by planting a seed or pruning a diseased part, but we know that whether it grows or heals is not our doing but a manifestation of its own expression of life. We can expect that each organism in an ecosystem, each cell within an organism has the capacity to 'get on with it'.

Living systems, of course, do more than just repair themselves, they continuously order themselves and maintain an identity. Not that they are conscious or have a *sense* of identity; but a tree, for example, maintains some sort of 'treeness' in a variety of different circumstances. The pattern and overall shape of a tree – the pattern of order of a tree – are exactly as one would expect them to be. But there is no way of predicting whether a particular location in space will be leaf, branch or air. The whole can be anticipated, nothing unexpected occurs, but the detail is nevertheless unpredictable.

Living systems are ordered but not controlled. DNA is sometimes described as a controller, a master molecule, but is in reality just one very important component of a complex chemical system.

The fact that people are *conscious* beings adds another dimension to the way human living systems work.

The metaphor of living systems

Web of relationships and communication

If you look at an organisation, or collection of organisations, using the metaphor of living systems, what would stand out? First, you would probably notice whether it struck you as 'alive' – the sort of impression you often get from first contacts. You would notice the quality of the relationships and the way that people are connected; whether conversations go beyond 'if you can't find it on the shelves, then we don't stock it'.

In a living system, each element is responsible for playing a part in the creation of other elements and of the system as a whole. This goes beyond simply the ability of one element to influence and respond to other elements – each has a responsibility to contribute to the functioning of other elements. Such a relationship is generative, it gives rise to growth or change in the other. The ability of an element to influence the system derives from the richness and strength of its connections.

You would also be aware of the formal power structure, the pyramidal organisation diagram, but in the foreground would be the connections, the 'informal' web of relationships and communication (Fig. 2). Some links are established and maintained formally. Others are established and maintained through informal networks.

Fig. 2 **Informal networks**

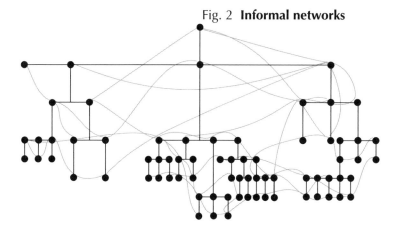

You would notice the people who are well connected, that others turn to and communicate with, who can be relied on to make the next link. You would notice where there is circularity in the web, where people can learn about the consequences of their actions, where there are feedback loops – for this is the fundamental pattern of organisation of life. The richness of these connections is essential if a human system is to avoid stasis or rigidity.

Not everybody needs to be connected to everybody else – just the relationships needed to do the job well and to catalyse change, the quality of reciprocity.

Many perspectives

If this web of connections and communication that makes up the informal system is the key to the life of the organisation, how can you use it most effectively? Low down the pyramid are people (including lay people, operational workers and middle managers) who may be *consulted* by those at the top of the formal power structure but who rarely have a chance to put things 'on the agenda' or to shape options. Organisations that function as living systems make use of the resourcefulness and perspectives of all these people. Such a system is so complex that no one person can have a complete picture of what goes on. In our experience the broadest picture is frequently held by lay people, who are particularly aware of the connections between different parts of the service. Including the perspective of lay people is not just some obligation borne by publicly funded services but an essential part of the workings of organisations functioning as living systems. The challenge is to find ways of drawing all these perspectives into the life of the organisation.

Meaning

People are purposeful and the meaning they attach to what they do is an important aspect of their individual identities. (This includes consciousness, unlike some other systems.) When people are able to act in a way that is congruent with their identity, they are able to act passionately.

If organisations are to function as living systems, they need shared purpose and meaning. Meaning gives coherence to the multitude of individual actions – sometimes expressed as the adage 'think global, act local'. Without shared (global) meaning individuals would not be able to organise their (local) work in a way that is both flexible and in tune with the system as a whole.

System that knows itself

'Who am I?' is a fundamental human question. Identity provides the basis for stability (homeostasis) and also for change. 'Who are we?' is a question that goes to the heart of any organisation or social group. These identities may be fluid, multiple and overlapping, and depend on meaning and purpose.

When we refer to a 'human system' we are not talking about something that is designed and maintained from outside – like the 'health care system', for example. Living systems exist to maintain their own identity. You know you are part of a human system not because 'I work for X' but because 'I feel part of Y'. A 'human system' assembles itself around a shared purpose – 'making this a good place to grow old in', for example. A human system does not have a fixed organisational structure but a pattern of connections and communications that occur over and over again.

A network of people may share a purpose even though this is not expressed or made explicit. They have an identity even if they are not consciously aware of it. Their opportunities are much greater if they recognise that they are playing a part in a living system. They may become aware not just of themselves and other elements, but of the boundaries of the system and the emergent properties of the system as a whole. This allows them to explore how their own behaviour affects the behaviour of the system as a whole. It allows them to go beyond simply doing their own bit well and enables them to hold themselves accountable for the behaviour of the system as a whole.

Participation

In a living system each element plays its part. If an organisation is to function as a living system, each individual and group are responsible for playing their part directly. The challenge is to find appropriate ways of going beyond consultation – simply inviting and giving advice and opinions. It is to find ways of working that encourage people to participate and to take responsibility together and not to rely on representatives to transmit opinions.

Trusting local resourcefulness

If an organisation, or network of organisations, functions as a living system, you would expect that this informal network would enable it to live, to 'keep on the move'. Each living system is unique and so the adaptive path it takes has to be appropriate to its unique circumstances. This organic capacity to adapt and change when necessary, without design and control by the formal system or by outsiders, is what we refer to as 'trusting local resourcefulness'.

Of course you often encounter human systems that are not behaving as you would like them to. We think that these systems are indeed being resourceful in their capacity to maintain their identity – but that the purpose, meaning and values around which they construct this identity are not those that you espouse. If one organisation is failing to work well with others, we would expect that its purpose and values differ from those of the other organisations and that it is doing what it can to maintain its own identity.

All organisations set out with a 'primary purpose' – what the organisation is trying to achieve. This might be maximising profit, for example, or providing a service of the highest possible quality. It will also have 'secondary purposes' – building capacity in the local community, for example, or providing job security for employees. When the going gets tough, surviving and maintaining the organisation's identity becomes critical. Often this manifests itself in resourceful maintenance of one or more of the organisation's secondary purposes, at the expense of the primary purpose.

Passion

Living systems are hungry – they need a source of energy to keep them alive. People choose to participate when they feel passionate about something. When organisations function as living systems they tap into this energy in a way that makes the energy available to the organisation and re-energises the individual or group.

Here and now

Living organisms may look messy, inefficient, and wasteful by comparison with mechanical systems. Millions of sperm are produced so that one can be available when needed. Ninety per cent of the brain doesn't have a 'job' name, but that doesn't mean it is doing nothing. Effectiveness in a living system is quite different from efficiency in a mechanical one.

A living system naturally operates in the here and now through multiple simultaneous processes. A living system must repair and renew itself, or die.

Patterns of order

Design and control have their place in organisations, but they are not required for order to emerge in living systems. Order in living systems shows itself both as stability and as the capacity to change.

Patterns of order emerge from the repeated application of a few simple rules. If human systems are similar, coherent patterns of order arise from a few principles that guide behaviour.

In summary ... In this chapter we consider two contrasting metaphors for the way organisations work. We are accustomed to using mechanical language and metaphor when we think about how organisations work. Whole system working uses instead the metaphor of a living system, or ecosystem, to understand the behaviour of organisations. This leads us to think of individuals, teams, departments, as purposeful, interdependent entities who can interact intelligently, autonomously and through a process of constantly adapting to each other. They are not limited to behaving in ways pre-determined by a designer. If you think of organisations as a living system, you pay attention to certain features such as connections, relationships and meaning. If you think of mechanical systems you pay attention to design, control mechanisms and so on.

Appendix: a theory of living systems

Underlying our experiential understanding of the nature of life are theories that describe and explain what it is. During the last quarter of a century growing numbers of biological scientists have taken an organismic rather than a mechanistic approach to the question 'what is life?' But while recognising living systems as qualitatively different from machines, they have not adopted the vitalist assertion that living systems involve some non-physical entity, force or field in addition to the familiar laws of physics and chemistry.

Organismic biologists, like vitalists, understand that the whole organism is more than the sum of its parts; but they recognise that this is a natural property of systems. The term 'emergent property' has been used since the 1920s to describe properties that emerge at a certain level of complexity but do not exist at lower levels – the wetness of water, for example, does not exist at the level of its atoms of hydrogen and oxygen. Life can be understood to be an emergent property of systems that have a certain level of complexity and are organised in a certain way. This organismic perspective has been described with particular clarity by Fritjof Capra in *The Web of Life*.

To appreciate this perspective it helps if we distinguish the 'structure' of an object from its 'pattern of organisation'. The pattern of organisation of a bicycle, for example, is a set of relationships between pedals and wheels, frame and handlebars. The pattern of organisation of a racing bike differs in small but significant ways (to do with ruggedness and drag) from the pattern of organisation of a mountain bike. The structure of a bike may be made of steel or aluminium, plastic or leather – different structures with the same pattern of organisation.

If you look at a standing wave set up when a stream flows over a rock, you have a choice whether you give attention to the structure (the particular molecules of water and rock present at that moment) or the pattern of organisation (the configuration of ordered relationships between its parts) that sustains the wave over the course of time. In the same way, whether thinking about an organism or a machine, it is possible to give attention to its pattern of organisation (the fundamental relationships and connections between its parts) or to its structure (the way that the pattern of organisation is embodied).

Structure

All living systems are 'open', in the sense that they are open to (and dependent on) energy and matter that flow through them. More than this, they have structures that are described as 'dissipative'. Living systems have important things in common with much simpler dissipative physical and chemical structures through which there is a flow of energy – for example, the vortex set up as a bath empties. If the flow of energy and matter ceases, such systems settle into equilibrium, or stasis. When this happens to a living system we describe it as 'dead'. Dissipative structures have the capacity to order themselves in stable yet dynamic ways under conditions that are far from equilibrium. You can reasonably expect that the bath-water will form a vortex of a certain size every time you pull out the plug, even though the detailed behaviour of the vortex – the intricacies of its shape and movement – is not predictable.

Pattern of organisation

The theory of autopoesis identifies the fundamental pattern of organisation of living systems as circularity. This occurs in the feedback loops that are to be found in networks. 'Living systems … [are] organised in a closed causal circular process that allows for evolutionary change in the way the circularity is maintained, but not for the loss of circularity itself'.

This organisational closure manifests itself in two particularly important ways. In the physical realm, the parts of the system are responsible for the circular pattern of organisation. Living systems are not inert but constantly remaking themselves, maintaining their integrity and renewing their elements. Each part must be produced and maintained by the other parts (not imported from outside) in order to maintain the circularity. 'Autopoesis' means 'self-making'.

In the realm of knowing, or cognition, perception is understood not as a representation of some external reality but as the constant creation of new relationships within a closed network.

For further reading, see page 161.

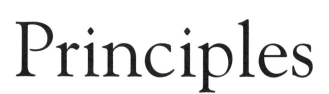

Principles

THE PRINCIPLES OF WHOLE SYSTEM
WORKING AND OUR EXPERIENCE
OF WHAT THEY MEAN IN PRACTICE

Whole system working is designed to help people make connections that enable them to find sustainable solutions to complex organisational problems. These connections are with both people and ideas. In this chapter we describe the principles which characterise this way of working, and our experience of putting them into practice.

We find it helpful to think about these as a constellation of ideas; each one matters and they are constantly moving in relation to each other. We have used the traditional device of a wheel to allow us to pay attention to one aspect at a time while keeping an awareness of the whole (see Fig. 3). This is the nearest we get to devising a sort of algorithm to describe the overall approach. Each aspect is important, but none is sufficient on its own. Bringing together people with many perspectives but no shared commitment, for example, may end up as a shouting match. Encouraging people to follow their passion without a sense of shared meaning may lead to just performance and posture.

Fig. 3 **Characteristics of whole system working**

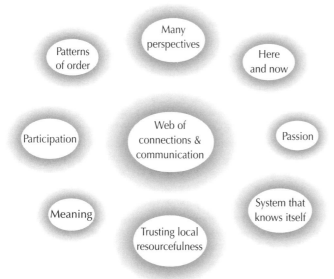

As you read on, you will recognise that whole system working is not a new invention. We think the living system metaphor (see page 14) describes what naturally goes on when communities and families are working well, but is rarely the way that organisations choose to work. You can make use of the whole system approach in many different circumstances and with groups of many different sizes. Sometimes large numbers of people use the approach together and we refer to these occasions as *whole system events*. These are not isolated events but highly visible moments in a much longer process. They enable people to become aware of being part of a wider system. This has a powerful symbolic effect, and brings the approach to the attention of lots of people. Because they provide some of the clearest illustrations of the approach in action, events appear frequently in the examples in this chapter.

None of the examples in this book describes single massive impacts, and in a sense they do not catch the quality of the approach at all. They describe details, particular meetings and specific actions. But each of these is part of a discernible pattern of:

- changing connections and access to relationships
- generating new flows of information
- explicit working with shared meaning in the sense of 'why we do things around here'.

The overall effect is substantial. We find that people struggle to express what they experience and they say things like the tangible changes are unremarkable but 'something' has changed in the way people relate to each other and organisations collaborate. It seems that the most significant impact of whole system working is on the 'health of the system'.

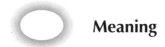

Meaning

All living systems exist to maintain their own identity.

In human systems, people are purposeful. Human systems come together around shared purpose and meaning.

Whole system working brings to the surface and makes available shared purpose and meaning.

We use the word 'system' to describe the people and organisations who connect around a shared purpose – an interest in neighbourhood safety, perhaps, or the quality of life of older people in a city. We do not use it in the sense of a formal organisational structure, such as the benefits system or the legal system. Clearly, in this 'informal' sense, people can choose to be part of many human systems and it is purpose and meaning that guide the choice.

Meaning and values and purpose are closely connected. We can think of purpose as the answer to the question, 'What?' (what are we trying to achieve?). We get at meaning through questions about 'Why?' (why are we trying to achieve this?). Values are abstractions that underlie meaning. Together they guide and order how individuals, and organisations, behave and prioritise their work (when not being coerced by external processes).

The purpose and values of an organisation are often encapsulated in a mission or vision statement. In a single organisation this may be drafted by people at the top, following consultative exercises, and the others are then encouraged to 'sign up' to the vision. By contrast, in a network where there is no 'top', purpose simply cannot be imposed. It has to be revealed in other ways. It is enough for people to understand each other's meaning. It is a bonus when they identify shared meaning. Working in ways that enable everyone to participate in finding common ground is the essence of the whole system approach. This is only possible if those in positions of power allow it to happen.

One of the pitfalls in discussions on meaning and purpose is that they tend to begin at a high level of abstraction. This excludes some people straightaway and tends to tidy up the richness of different viewpoints so we design and use methods that encourage people to begin with stories of real experience. We use dialogue as a specific way of working and we ensure that both lay people and people from many levels within organisations are part of the process.

By dialogue we mean a way of working in which different views are expressed, and assumptions explored as a means to discover a new view. This contrasts with discussion in which each person is usually trying to have his or her argument accepted by others: parts of other people's arguments may be accepted but the aim is usually to win.

One method of accessing stories is to ask people to work in pairs to share an experience that each of them has had about the issue in question. We bring together these accounts to show how things can be when the system operates at its best and then participants draw up a set of 'audacious propositions' that are both aspirational and grounded in real experience. These propositions describe how things could be in the future and they frequently illuminate what really matters to people, the meaning that underlies their actions.

Often when people are meeting around some burning local issue, the temptation to jump into problem-solving is overwhelming. We have learned that it pays handsomely to spend as much time as possible exploring purpose and possibilities. In our early site work we found that towards the end of long whole system events, participants were itching to get on to action and problem-solving and felt held back by the design of the meeting. We responded, in the next few meetings, by moving the action-planning to an earlier and longer time slot. These meetings were less successful – they were not able to come up with anything more than ideas their members already had in mind when they arrived. In other words, we had not allowed enough time for people to explore the possibilities offered by working in groups containing a completely new range of perspectives.

Sometimes people from different organisational cultures or different professions find it hard to 'hear' and respect the values of another group and reaching agreement on common ground is not an easy task. And within an overall sense of purpose there are many shades of interpretation and many different priorities that it is helpful to acknowledge. But if the overarching aim is to get people to behave in different ways, then it is necessary to 'hear' and respect the purpose, beliefs and values held by others.

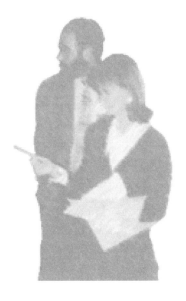

> ### *The purpose and values of others*
>
> People who suffer from chronic skin conditions rely on the skills and advice of many people – their GP, practice nurse, specialist nurses and doctors, pharmacists, other patients and their families, self-help groups and so on.
>
> A group of 30 managers, general practitioners, hospital specialists and specialist nurses spent a day together trying to agree an appropriate package of care for people with skin problems. Each tended to defend the priorities of their professional group. Fortunately, the participants also included people with skin problems, and one of them was able to say, 'We need you all, so you have to find a way of working together on this'.
>
> By bringing to attention their common purpose of caring for the individual patient these professionals were able to reach agreement about their respective contributions. It takes time to listen to each other – not something that can generally be achieved in a committee meeting with a full agenda – and it is no accident that this meeting lasted all day.

When people discover areas of shared purpose this allows them to choose to identify with the human system that operates around that purpose. They may even be able to see the functioning of this system as more important than the functioning of their organisation alone.

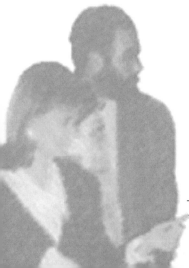

In this together

In one local site where people had been developing a whole system approach for some time, the local authority made a decision to cut the community care budget for the next financial year which would have knock-on effects on other agencies. They announced this the day before an important inter-agency meeting of about 25 senior people. Those from the NHS trusts, the health authority and the voluntary organisations expressed their disappointment, but with wry looks and an understanding that those from the local authority were in reality as disappointed as they were. Afterwards, people from health said they were surprised they had been able to have a constructive meeting in the circumstances; and those from the local authority were surprised that they had not been forced into defending the local authority decision.

Reconnecting with meaning can work in other ways too. It is easy for people to lose sight of the reason why their organisation exists, its primary purpose. In times of pressure priority may be given increasingly to secondary purposes, such as providing professional satisfaction, a tolerable working environment or just employment. Building a shared understanding of the purpose of an organisation, or network of organisations, allows people to reconnect with their primary purpose. This is not just an abstraction. It leads to shared commitment among those who choose to engage with it. There is no need to 'motivate' or 'empower' people when the energy is theirs. Some of this energy probably comes from the reduction in dissonance between what is said and what is done.

I think whole system working helps to put the purpose back into the work we do. I remember a group that moved away from its task at one of its meetings and ended up as a rich discussion of values – something organisations don't encourage you to talk about. One woman described how she had been troubled by something where she worked that she felt was 'not right', but that she had lost the energy and impetus to do anything about it. After discussing it in the group and getting support from them she felt able to go back and 'do battle'. I saw this as her regaining her sense of purpose. (Voluntary organisation manager)

 # System that knows itself

A living system knows itself in its environment.
It acts to conserve its identity.

If human systems know something of themselves as a whole within their environment, they have new opportunities.

Whole system working is an approach that enables people to recognise some of the human systems to which they belong by virtue of their commitment to shared purpose.

Most people operate as part of lots of human systems, and these change over time. A network of people with shared purpose has an identity, though they may not be consciously aware of it. When they recognise themselves as part of an interconnected system then the possibilities for action alter.

Human systems are about behaviour, the dynamic, circular, repeated patterns of connections and communication that allow us to adapt and evolve. What matters is how the people who are the parts of the system connect, act, behave and contribute to purpose. The system is best described by its behaviour, rather than its people.

Living systems organise themselves, constantly. If you are interested in changing the way a system operates, then you have to find ways of helping it to 'know itself', to be consciously aware of its purpose and its boundaries and the repeated interplay of its intentions and actions.

One rapid and graphic way of revealing connections is to pass a ball of string among a group of people, with each person passing it to someone with whom they have links. This soon reveals a tangle of interconnections. Another method we use to help the system know itself is to encourage groups of about 20–30 people to produce a system map together (see page 84 and page 126). Once again this is about uncovering and revealing connections and pathways. Most people learn something they didn't know before and we are constantly impressed by how energising this exercise can be. The first time we used it, we worked with a group of operational managers in a district hospital and their 'significant contacts' in the borough. We had reservations about whether this mixed group would find the exercise engaging, let alone useful, and were astonished how powerful they found it, and how people still remember it three years later.

Geography and scale of operation are other factors which help people recognise whether they are part of a particular system or not. We have applied whole system working to geographical areas as small as a general practice catchment area and as large as a city. Getting clear about purpose is the other factor that really matters in making the system visible to itself. When people recognise others who want to work on the same issue as they do, it can be inspirational. When someone realises that a particular group has a purpose which is different from theirs, then they leave and avoid wasting their time.

Getting clear about purpose

A group of about a dozen people wanted to do something about transport for elderly people. They came from several organisations including the ambulance service. After a while, it became clear that their real concern was about the buses. This allowed the ambulance service to withdraw, but the contacts and connections had begun and were there for future use.

Another powerful way of helping the system 'to know itself' is literally to see the diversity of people in one room together. This can begin as soon as a few unlikely people get together and is most apparent in whole system events with large numbers of people. Generating a sense of 'all being in this together' can liberate energy to re-engage with long-standing issues. The significant value added by these methods of working is the extra energy released when the responsibility for solution-finding belongs to everybody. At one meeting of 170 people an elderly woman was taken aback by the numbers present : 'I never realised there were this many people in the city who cared about older people.'

Once the system is aware of itself, people and organisations improve their ease of access to each other because they understand their interdependence. They put faces to names. They develop confidence about who they can telephone. They find their way around more easily and seek information in new ways. Simply being present at a meeting is not in itself enough to allow this to happen. But when participants have understood each others' purpose and the web of connections that support it they seem to recognise that they are part of the same system. They may also recognise the possibility of acting consciously as a whole.

It was good to find out what other people are doing. A lot of people have no idea of what the others are doing, for example in voluntary organisations. I think it was brilliant to work and meet people from different backgrounds.
(Worker, Community & Leisure Services)

We really needed something like that. I have found the whole process very interesting. I think I can understand what other organisations are doing. I can find my way around much better now. (Manager, Passenger Transport Authority)

 ## Many perspectives

In a living system each element has its own identity which contributes to the identity of the whole. These identities, separate and overlapping, provide the variety and redundancy necessary for adaptation. They provide a range of choices and reduce the risk of catastrophic failure.

If a human system is similar, the presence of many perspectives is an essential resource. By contrast the search for one correct perspective reduces the capacity to adapt.

The challenge of whole system working is to find processes which exploit different ways of seeing things and make them available for use.

Our beliefs about cause and effect and how the world works influence what we do and what we imagine we could do. They structure the way we perceive reality. The reason they matter is that we act according to our individual mental maps. Therefore if we want to find new ways of working we need to find new mental maps. There are lots of these around.

Each person has a rather different mental map. For instance, in a single organisation, such as a hospital, the mental maps that are held by porters, nurses, doctors, managers, patients and visitors will be different. Each group, and within each group each individual, will see different things about what is important in this organisation and how it works.

We sometimes refer to long-standing, 'messy' problems as 'elephant problems' – not because they are grey and immovable but as a reference to the Sufi proverb about blind men examining an elephant. Each can feel one part – the tail, the trunk, the legs. Each has his own understanding of one part of the elephant – his own 'mental map'.

You may reasonably expect that an expert, perhaps the chief executive of your organisation, is able to see the 'big picture'. But this 'big picture' is a single perspective and lacks a lot of very important detail. The chief executive knows a lot about the organisation from reports and conversations. He recognises the importance of the experience and wisdom of his employees and may have found formal ways to make use of this through specific structures (e.g. quality circles). He listens to the views of customers, clients or patients through consultation, market research and consumer satisfaction appraisal (questionnaires, surveys and focus groups) as well as listening to complaints and analysing critical incidents. Yet he may have little idea about the quality of the conversations between junior nurses and patients' relatives, though this may be one of the most important things that determine whether people find their stay in hospital satisfactory.

If this is the case for a single organisation, how much more so for the many different organisations that influence the quality of a stay in hospital. How is it possible to get the 'big picture' that includes relatives, neighbours, district nurses, ambulances, general practitioners, taxis, interpreters, home helps and many more – as well as numerous hospital staff? The approach we describe is not a search for the overview but a way of making use of the understanding that there are lots of 'part' views. The question is not whether, but how, the many perspectives can be accommodated; how the understanding and experience of different sorts of people can contribute to change. We are not looking for overlap or consensus, though they are important, but for the emergence of new insights that help the whole system to adapt.

The practical task of working from a whole system perspective is to provide methods of working which not only identify and bring together a rich variety of perspectives but enable the people who hold them to work together constructively. This is not about being nice to each other, it is about accessing a system-wide resource.

Hearing other perspectives

Starting to work from a whole system perspective means thinking about and finding unusual mixes of people each of whom contributes another mental map. We use the word system to mean something that assembles itself around a shared purpose. What is the right mix of people for that purpose and how do their voices get heard? We don't have a recipe for the 'right' mix but we do know that diversity is the key. Yet when people from diverse backgrounds come together on some issue they feel strongly about, they may be hindered not just by feelings but by different styles of communication. In our experience, methods which work successfully here pay attention to three factors:

- careful use of time
- people work from experience and everyone's expertise is used
- conversation is the unit of currency and much work gets done in small groups, no matter how many people take part overall.

One local government director summed up his experience of encountering new mental maps by reading out a quote from Ishiguro's novel, *The Remains of the Day*:

I have never in all these years thought of the matter in quite this way; but then it is perhaps in the nature of coming on a trip such as this that one is prompted towards such surprising new perspectives on topics one imagined one had long ago thought through thoroughly.

Sometimes there is a history of misunderstanding or conflict between agencies, or of antagonism from lay people who feel they have been 'consulted to death' but never listened to. Where there is long-standing neglect or oppression of a group of people, it may simply be another form of oppression to ask them to discuss constructively the future before they have had an opportunity to express their anger. In situations like these whole system working requires preparatory work that permits the expression of anger and frustration, and builds a shared experience of listening and being listened to. There are many ways of doing this and all involve hearing how things really are. This requires, at the very least, enough time for people to have their say and recognise that they have been heard – in public. One of the things we work to avoid is professionals being put in the position of having to defend their organisation's behaviour, of having to stick to the 'official line' and fight their corner.

Tackling existing conflict and misunderstanding

In one of the places we have been working, the 'winter bed crisis' of the previous year had left a legacy of recrimination between general practice, the hospital, the health authority and the social services department as well as a sense of insecurity among local residents, particularly elderly people. Everyone wanted to avoid a repetition the following year but it seemed hard for them to begin co-operating without first dealing with the bad feelings still around.

Before meeting to explore the possibilities for the future, we encouraged them to revisit the past. One hundred and forty people sat at round tables in a large room. They were arranged in 'likeness' groups – general practice together, social services together, elderly residents together and so on.

Each group explored their own perspective of the previous year's 'winter bed crisis' and prepared a three-minute story they could tell everybody in the room. They were asked to tell the story honestly, and to be clear that they were describing not 'the truth' but their own view, using words like 'we believed that...' and 'it seemed to us that ...'

People were asked to listen with the intention of understanding the viewpoints of others – not to discover the truth or get the facts right, but to listen for surprises where other people's viewpoint was different from their own. They were asked to listen for how their role was perceived by others, recognising these perceptions might make them angry or upset. They were not asked to respond to what sounded like criticism or to 'set the record straight' but to ask themselves what led to these perceptions. They used this understanding to make posters that showed to the others how we think we are seen/how we would like to be seen/ what we would need to do to be seen in this way. Each group who had had 'their say' could tell whether the others had heard by looking at the posters.

> *The poster work was an incredible shock to many people. Users were seen as the cause of the problem. The voluntary sector saw the statutory bodies as asleep. The local authority (mainly social services) drew themselves as in the stocks. Everybody was very angry with the council ... Since then people have spent a lot of time talking about it.* (Senior manager)

After lunch the participants were able to work together in a very co-operative atmosphere. The plans they began to formulate have since led to significant improvement in local services.

Sometimes a most powerful tool is the ability of professionals to really listen and to feed back what they have heard. And yet there are many factors which limit this. Professionals may actually feel irresponsible acknowledging things they hear but cannot do anything about. Appropriately enough, they find it easiest to acknowledge what they have heard when they are in a position to analyse the problem and do something about it. To the person expressing important views without getting any response, however, it may feel as though the professionals have not been listening. Whole system working deliberately uses techniques for listening, and recording, in public which can be an extremely useful means of moving discussions on in a spirit of honesty. Participants can see their words written on the wall and used as the agenda. And one of the things we have learned in practice is that capturing the exact words matters. We once tried to be helpful and typed up the words from a set of flipcharts, grouped them, and returned them to the people who had produced them. They treated what was written on these sheets of paper as though they had been imposed arbitrarily from outside. Tidying up material sometimes loses all the power of the original, which can still convey the energy and quality of the conversations of which it is a summary.

How things really are

We were asked to plan a meeting that would explore what people wanted during the course of an urban regeneration programme. The development had been under way for some time and had proved to be very disruptive. It included 'decanting' local residents from their homes while new houses were built. Local elderly people were suspicious of the development partnership, and residents had resorted to legal action to halt the building work on the grounds that the promised consultation had not taken place. Professional expectation was extremely low and nervous. They expected very few people to come to the meeting, or, if they did, to be uncooperative and make unreasonable demands.

We designed a meeting with the aim of getting elders and professionals to understand each other's points of view a bit better than before – a simple but fundamental step. In the event 120 people, including 90 elders, turned out to 'Speak your mind'. They worked in mixed groups of eight at round tables discussing 'How do we build a good place to grow old in?', and then fed back their views to the whole room using a roving microphone. As these views were expressed, the facilitators wrote their words on a 'public listening wall' and publicly sorted them into themes. Participants then chose one of these themes for their afternoon's work.

At the end of the day a few participants from the agencies were asked to tell everybody what they had heard. One of these was the chair of the development partnership who said he had intended to stay for one hour but had then decided to stay for the day. He had changed his mind when he found not confrontation but 'older people who have ideas about their community, are passionate about the future, and are willing and able to get involved'.

A significant feature of this design was that professionals were asked not to provide solutions or 'to fix' problems, and not to make any promises. Instead, they were asked to listen and to feed back what they had heard. Older people felt better that they had got their concerns and interests across and they were realistic about what could and could not be addressed. The evaluation shows that this day was viewed positively by almost all those interviewed.

After this meeting an elders partnership group, made up of local residents and professionals from several agencies, contributed actively to two of the themes that had been highlighted at the meeting – the development of the town centre and access to health care.

Working with diversity

Finding constructive ways of working with diversity is one of the most significant aspects of whole system working. Once it is clear that there is a system-wide issue (i.e. not a problem that would be better dealt with by an individual organisation) and that the system wants to tackle it (i.e. not just one particular profession or one agency), then the language which is used to describe the issue becomes critical, because that is the way people recognise whether it matters to them, or not. In other words, the way the issue is described allows people to identify whether they are part of the system. It expresses shared meaning and thus sets the boundary for that particular system.

Finding the right people to join in becomes the next critical step. In this context 'right' means a sufficiently mixed group to support new connections, combinations and possibilities. It is the sufficient mix that matters whether numbers are small or large. Diversity is always important but when you get to working with large numbers of people the opportunities are even greater. We have learned from experience that the mix of people must include:

- different levels within an organisation and across organisations – frontline staff and directors of strategy, operators and board members, clients and middle managers

- people who know how 'to connect' and are interested in doing things differently – the people who can make things happen (some of whom may be 'troublesome'), the sort of people whose support makes it likely that others will follow, as well as those with formal power

- lay people or clients or customers – their perspective is essential and often missing

- people with continuing relationships and repeated interactions – if there is no commitment to future interaction then bringing people together gives you an ark, a sample of each kind, not a system.

Twenty per cent at least

We have learned that the participation of lay people is essential. Much of our work has been about services for older people and in one place the phrase No Elders, No Meeting became a kind of mantra.

We have also learned that the proportion of lay people in a whole system event is critical. At least 20 per cent of participants have to be service users, citizens, clients, customers. Their perspective is no more 'right' than any other but their voice often makes it easier for professionals to reach agreement on meaning – whatever secondary purposes an organisation acquires, its primary purpose is usually to provide goods or services to lay people. And the active participation of lay people helps professionals hang on to a sense of 'the whole', which is no easy task.

In one of the early events we designed, the planning group was confident that local people would respond well to an invitation to take part. The lead agency was rightly proud of its good relations with its service users and so when they were building the invitation list the planning group's efforts went in other directions. The result was disappointing. Not enough lay people took part and the agenda was captured by the professionals present. Although some good ideas were advanced, the event did not give rise to the usual rich inventiveness.

From a whole system perspective, working with diversity is about finding new assets, not new problems. People begin to see reality differently and this can lead to different understanding which is a necessary precursor to different action. When a mixed group work well together, they treat each other respectfully as interdependent collaborators. They want to produce something together. This seems to make them more aware of situations where this respect is missing and keen to spread this way of working.

 ## Participation

In a living system one of the responsibilities of every element is to fulfil its own function.

If a human system is similar, each individual or group is responsible for playing its part directly. This cannot be done for them or on their behalf. Each part is necessary.

Whole system working requires the direct participation of those involved.

Whole system working is about each person, team, department, agency playing its part. All are needed and everyone is asked to participate as an individual, and not as a representative of a community or profession or organisation. Most people's experience of taking part in interagency work is rather different.

If the purpose of the meeting is monitoring or audit, for example, and someone from the police is invited they will almost certainly be expected to represent the formal power structure of the police. If there have been problems, they will be expected to 'take it on the chin' when their organisation comes in for criticism and to transmit that criticism, when appropriate, up the formal power structure, to provide a mechanism for holding the organisation accountable for past behaviour. They will be expected to respond on behalf of the organisation by providing explanations or apologies and by making commitments about how the organisation will behave in the future. They will therefore have to contribute tactfully, portray their own organisation in the best possible light, even when they personally disapprove of how it has behaved, and avoid making any rash promises that others in the organisation will not be happy with.

On the contrary, if the purpose of the meeting is to explore possibilities, as it is when you work from a whole system perspective, then the design is such that participants are not put in this position. You may decide that you want to invite the police but the person who comes will be asked to contribute their own point of view, and will neither be held to account for the behaviour of 'the police' nor be expected to make commitments on their behalf. We design meetings in ways that people may hear criticism of their organisation, and may even have to acknowledge that they have heard what has been said, but they are never asked to justify publicly past behaviour. They may choose to make a personal commitment to some course of action in the future, but they are not asked to make commitments for their organisation. The personal commitment may, of course, involve the organisation – 'I will invite a lay person on to this committee' if that is in their power, or 'I will ask my manager if I can do so' if it is not. These individual actions take place in the informal network rather than the formal power structure (see page 15).

What matters from a whole system perspective is everyone's personal responsibility as a participant. Simply being present is not enough.

When you invite people to participate as individuals, they sometimes find it hard to believe, or even to understand what you mean. We have found it helpful to think of three different forms of engagement: visitor, complainant, and co-producer (these are derived from therapist–client relationship in solution-based therapy). Those who have a *visitor relationship* attend because they have been invited or sent, not because they have any expectation that a solution can be found. Those who have a *complainant relationship* attend because they can identify a complaint that they want addressed. They see their responsibility as clearly articulating the complaint while it is the responsibility of somebody else to come up with a solution. Those who have a *co-producer relationship* want to take responsibility for finding a solution in the company of others.

People who engage as visitors may initially be sceptical but get rapidly drawn into the participatory co-producing relationship. Those who describe themselves as cynical or hostile at the outset usually remain so.

People who engage as complainants are good at articulating their concerns. They may derive some of their legitimacy from the fact that they represent a wider constituency, for example, a campaigning group. They often encounter the whole system approach expecting the sort of consultation exercise for which they are so well prepared. Some find the approach disturbing, unsatisfactory and 'undemocratic'. Others, seizing the opportunity to participate, find it liberating and adopt a co-producing relationship. Whole system working relies on people recognising their ability to become interdependent co-producers of new solutions to local concerns.

What whole system working can do is to allow people to surface what it is they are willing to collaborate on – the so-called common ground – and to start to generate the connections and information flows that can sustain it. A group of people do what that group of people choose to do and are capable of doing. They may take insights and requests to and from their communities, but they do so as individuals, not as

representatives. They are not asked to commit their organisation or community to anything, just to commit themselves.
Whole system working is not about campaigning to change
the behaviour of others outside the group (important though
campaigning may be in appropriate circumstances). It is about
'what we can do together'. Of course, the 'we' who are present
may not be enough to do anything. It may be necessary to ask
'who else do we need to involve?' and 'how are we to engage
them?' and that in turn means more connections and more
sharing of purpose and so on.

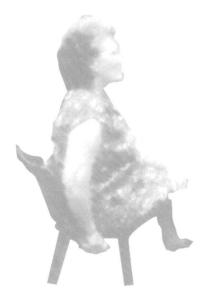
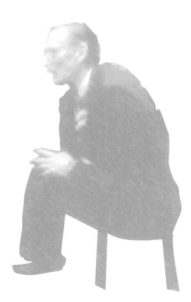

What can we do together?

One group of 10–20 got together because they wanted to do something about improving transport for older people. There was a strong nucleus of elders, people from the voluntary sector, the police and a transport company. Initially, the struggle was to find a way of using the strengths of this unusual membership. The group first tried to act as if it were able to represent older people and hold those in the formal system to account. We encouraged them to identify something they could all work on together and they decided on bus services. Recognising that bus drivers had a shared interest in this they focused on the question 'how can we enable bus drivers to provide the service that older people want?'

Several older people, with experience of getting things done by campaigning, wanted the group to campaign to persuade the bus company to schedule longer journey times, to allow more time for passengers to sit down, to go back to two-crew bus operations and to extend the hours of the concessionary bus pass.

If the group had taken this approach, the bus operators and police would have left. We kept emphasising the word 'we', and the fact that the potential in a whole system group lies in doing things that all those who identify with that system can get done together. Those who wanted to campaign identified another forum where they could continue to do so.

By retaining the identity of a system containing many perspectives the group discovered that what they could productively do together was for older people and managers from the bus companies to travel together on the buses and share their experiences. This led to improved understanding by the older people of the bus operators. It also led to a recognition by the managers that older people are a resource who have useful things to say about bus design and operation. As a result, they immediately put into effect some inexpensive but significant modifications to the buses; took the comments of the older people into the driver training programme; and invited older people to view and assess new buses they were thinking of buying.

There are lots of participative working methods that enable people to contribute constructively from personal experience. We have found that apparently minor detail counts every bit as much as the design of the meeting. We use round tables for easy and equal conversation, for instance. We use ground rules for small discussion groups that encourage all to contribute; name badges without titles; roving microphones that enable everyone in a large group to comment, not just those used to speaking in public. People become more confident as a result. The information that is publicly recorded on the walls of the room is a common resource and, as it builds up, there is no way of telling who contributed which bit.

In most of the examples we describe lay people have played a central role, and this is recognised by all those who have been involved. Sometimes they go on to greater things – part of the solution and not the problem.

Part of the solution not the problem

In one borough social services managers have engaged and paid a group of elders to help assess the quality of standards in residential homes. In another, elders have been recruited, trained and paid to conduct interviews for two research programmes into sexual health and hospital discharge. In both instances there was a feeling that the elders who had been interviewed felt more comfortable than they would have with younger interviewers.

A whole system group that wanted to improve Leisure, Pleasure and Learning recognised that elderly people were discouraged from taking part in fitness activities led by young people at their peak of fitness. They wanted to train elders to become fitness trainers themselves. They succeeded in raising some £12,000 and provided courses for 20 elders, several of whom are now employed in local leisure centres.

Often it is the ability of lay people to engage through personal experience, rather than generalisation, that is particularly valuable. Getting used to the power of stories can change professional behaviour in ways which are long-lasting. Two years after taking part in a whole system event on the quality of life for older people, interviewees from a range of background thought it had led to significant changes in attitude.

At a meeting of the older people's JPT [joint planning team] two of the older people's representatives were noticeably upset. Their distress was caused by their personal situations and concern about the circumstances of other older people known to them. At first it seemed that the meeting would sympathetically listen to these personal anecdotes – but regard them as having no general relevance, certainly not to admit them as evidence of more widespread system failures – and then carry on with its business. But Mr K from the health authority stepped in and supported the older people. He agreed to their suggestion that time should be given at each meeting for the airing of personal stories – from anyone. This was quite a dramatic intervention. There was nearly dissension in the statutory ranks. But others rallied to support Mr K, and it was widely discussed and agreed. This was a critical point where something suddenly shifted.
(Local authority manager)

At one time I would have been only 'business-orientated'. If two older people had got upset, I would have been impatient to get on with the meeting – I would never have seen their concerns as the legitimate business of the meeting. I've become more tolerant and prepared to take more risk.
(Health authority manager)

Service planners and providers always find it very difficult to hear these stories. They don't want to hear them. They have to deny them or rule them out of order as mere anecdotes, not hard evidence. For to accept the elders' stories as true would mean having to confront things and admit that they are not as they – the funders and providers – present them. This is very threatening. So to get stories allowed is a small triumph. But the crunch has to come in what happens as a result of what people say. (Voluntary agency director)

There are already small changes in services as a result of elders' stories. For example, there will be changes to security in sheltered housing as a result of an anecdote described at a planning meeting. The manager came along to the next meeting and we all discussed it. (Voluntary sector worker)

Web of connections and communication

In living systems the elements are responsible for contributing to the function of other elements as well as fulfilling their own function. There is a web of connections and the behaviour of the elements is co-ordinated by the communication that flows through feedback loops in the web.

If a human system is similar, the parts are linked in a web of connections and communication. Each part is responsible not only for their own function, but also for contributing to the functioning of other parts and thus to the whole.

Whole system working reveals and supports networks of connections and the communications that sustain them.

In living systems the capacity to get things done is distributed widely, not in just a few skilled operators. Building networks of personal contacts is part of the job. This is not about good personal relationships but an essential characteristic of how living, or adaptive, systems function. In order to play their part people need to be able to call upon others, when necessary, and the flow of communication has to be circular. The feedback loops have to work. Connections and information flows are an essential part of being effective, not an optional gloss, and when a system is 'stuck' or not functioning well, this is one of the characteristics that has to be brought to attention.

> *In the old days when something needed to be done in this city I could get on the phone to half-a-dozen people and it would get done. Nowadays it's not so simple.* (Local authority director)

Connections and relationships grow from opportunities to share experiences and explore what we mean and to be able to do so repeatedly, not just in one-off activity. In human systems, sharing experience is almost always about language. Whole system working allows enough time for conversations to build connections. The work is designed to ensure that these conversations are rooted in personal experience, not generalisation. We have learned that the size of a group is critical if people are to work productively and that round tables enable people to hear each other, no matter how many are in the room altogether. Round tables are not about seating arrangements – that's where the work gets done.

There are lots of ways of drawing out connections and helping people recognise the links between them and how well they operate. One way is to build up a map together (see page 84 and page 126). Another may be, literally, getting people in the room together around a common concern. Generating a sense of 'all being in this together' can liberate energy but only if the meeting is about engaging with purpose – what is it we care about here? In human systems it is purpose or meaning that ultimately decides the level of energy people are prepared to commit.

> *Participants … invariably said that in some intangible way things were beginning to happen but they would be hard-pressed to give tangible evidence to support that claim. There is a clear sense that people have a much better understanding*

of the informal networks (i.e. who to call on and for what problem) that need to be leveraged in order for substantial change to occur. Nevertheless, many of the participants in the events pointed out that these subtle changes in behaviour cannot be easily measured. (Evaluator, McKinsey & Company)

Often we value most highly the relationships we have with people who are similar to ourselves. We are comfortable making connections with 'people like us' and we can tell if we are in the 'right place' by the other people in the room. In several of the places we have worked, board-level people arrive for a meeting, find there is nobody else of equivalent seniority present, and leave before the meeting begins. But where leaders reach out beyond this pattern, either within their own organisation or across other organisations, it is always noticed and always makes a difference. Our experience is that where whole system working flourishes, there are several senior people prepared to make this stretch.

Another thing that happens is that people can see more easily how to contribute to the functioning of other parts of the system.

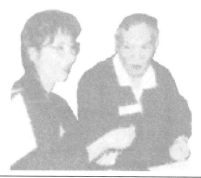

Contributing to other parts of the system

One of the 'classic' boundary issues in the Health Service is when people get admitted to hospital, and when they leave hospital to return home. For most people most of the time it works. But it can be a disaster of misinformation and lack of co-ordination. Communication between GPs and hospitals is crucial. In one of the places we worked, a group of GPs knew the importance of a really good 'admission letter' to ensure that their local hospital got all the information it needed when a patient was admitted, and they had worked hard to produce a good format. During the course of a whole system event they realised that, no matter how good the letter was, the hospital was not able 'to hear' what they were communicating because of the way junior hospital doctors rotate between departments. In other words, they realised that if they wanted to get their message across, and to influence what the hospital actually did, they would have to become involved in the hospital's induction programme for doctors. And this they set about doing.

What happened during the whole system event was that the GPs surfaced and respected the fact that, as well as treating individual patients, hospitals have the additional purpose of training junior doctors. This enabled them to move on to different action to achieve their goal.

At some level, of course, everyone 'knows' that hospitals train junior staff but that does not mean this knowledge can be acted upon. Further evidence of reciprocal relationships would be if the hospital were able to respect the GPs' additional purpose of continuing care for patients and supply really helpful discharge letters.

Trusting local resourcefulness

A living system with its environment has the capacity to adapt.

*If a human system is similar, it too has within it
the capacity to adapt and change, and need not
depend on external design and control.*

*Whole system working is an approach that trusts that
local people, groups and organisations can be sufficiently
resourceful to adapt appropriately without
the need for external design.*

Living systems will order themselves and manage their own activities. Stable patterns of order will emerge. Our understanding of a living system is that its pattern of organisation is produced within the system itself. This cannot be directly changed from outside, although the system is not unresponsive to changes in its environment. Living systems exist at the edge of equilibrium, an interesting place where stable patterns of order arise but where there is also the capacity to adapt and change.

If a living system is behaving not as you would like, this is probably because it is ordering itself very effectively around meaning and purpose that you do not share.

When organisations and networks of organisations function as living systems, they have within them the capacity to adapt. The resources necessary for change may be identified within the system itself in the form of new people, new flows of information, new passion or new connections. (There are many situations where human systems need *more* resources but often energy and resources are consumed just to maintain the status quo.)

Recognising capacities

People, and organisations, are not always aware of their own capacities. Bringing these to attention is an important part of whole system working, which we describe as asset-based (i.e. recognising capacities and exploring possibilities) in contrast to deficit-based approaches (i.e. recognising deficiencies and trouble-shooting problems). There is no reason to confine interventions to one end of this range. Sometimes simply bringing to attention the assets in a group is enough to allow them to recognise what they have and what they want to do.

Recognising capacities

A small group of older people got together to promote life-long learning. When a new member joined, they decided to spend some time itemising useful contacts, skills and interests.

Initially, some members felt that they might have little to contribute but within a few minutes the pens and pencils were scribbling away.

We were members of local, regional, national and international organisations designed to provide service to communities locally and globally. We were governors of schools; we served on public bodies. One of us was a highly accomplished linguist with a professional background in translation and interpretation. Age had not diminished our athleticism – we climbed, fell walked, trampolined and swam. We exercised our brains with antique hunting, creative writing, music and the arts. And we hadn't forgotten future generations; several members spent time working with children and recording reminiscences. What a wealth of knowledge and expertise was there.

It seemed only a small step for them to decide to organise an activity-led summer school for local older people, which they set about doing.

When we focus on positive images of the future, we increase the likelihood that such a future will come about. We all recognise this when we use phrases like the 'self-fulfilling prophecy'. Our own positive images can influence our future as we know from the placebo effect and the techniques used by athletes to visualise success. The positive images others have of us can also influence our future, for instance, when a teacher believes that a student has greater than average potential the student invariably does better. Our images of ourselves are held in our own inner dialogue. The image of a human system, a business or city perhaps, is held in the stories we tell each other about it.

We can choose to dwell on narratives that are energy-diminishing or energy-enhancing, to see the glass as half-empty or half-full. The choice we make about the stories we tell of what happens around us has the potential to change behaviour now, and to influence the way the future unfolds.

In places where people are beginning to work with a whole system approach they may start by celebrating successes, particularly achievements or talents that are taken for granted. Instead of asking why something goes wrong, we can choose instead to ask what the conditions are when it goes right – instead of looking at the problem of cities, we can ask what makes a well-functioning city work. This has been called 'taking an appreciative stance', in the sense of artistic appreciation which may not be uncritical but has less to do with apportioning blame and more to do with curiosity and a desire to understand. Work processes can be designed that enable good people to do things well (rather than simply stopping poor people from doing things badly). Seeking out energy-generating moments can include experiences which cause intense frustration or distress as well as success and these can all produce insights into things we care passionately about.

However, this way of working does have to be approached with some caution, especially when people have anger and frustration that they need to express. We have found professionals in the NHS reacting with suspicion to a request to describe any positive experience unless they have first had the opportunity to express the negative.

Taking an appreciative stance

In one borough there was concern to find out how to improve the quality of people's experience of being in the local hospital. The NHS professionals in the group found it difficult to ask about positive stories, or acknowledge them when they found any.

One person told about Mrs J who had established really successful telephone communication with the ward when her mother was an inpatient. All those who heard this story discounted it because Mrs J was 'special'. She was a physiotherapist, and communication tends to be easier when a person has 'inside' knowledge of the NHS.

Yet poor telephone communication between relatives and hospital wards is a well-recognised problem which never seems to get fixed, however much effort is put into dealing with complaints.

The group realised that it might be productive to pay great attention to the factors that enable health professionals to establish good communication, and to find ways of generalising from them to all relatives.

Self-managing abilities

Our experience is that using asset-based techniques develops the capacity of people to manage their own activities. They become increasingly confident that this can result in activity which produces outcomes. For this to happen the self-managing has to be 'bounded', particularly by a sense of purpose – what is it we care about here – and by some practical processes.

Working at 5ft round tables enables eight people to work together. The groups manage the work themselves, whatever the task. There is no group facilitator but we encourage them to adopt the roles of timekeeper, recorder, reporter and discussion leader. Using these as 'ground rules,' self-managing groups create a variety of ways of working. Sometimes they effortlessly rotate roles as suggested. Sometimes one person takes the lead and the others go along with it. Sometimes they adopt formal committee-style behaviour. Sometimes they flounder.

Our experience of whole system events where there are perhaps 20 tables of eight people in the same room is that sometimes a table appears to be unable to find a way of working and gives up. Sometimes groups are very productive, but not in the ways the organisers intended. Sometimes they just go round and round in circles. Sometimes they are both painful and unhelpful. We have found that dysfunctional groups are much less likely when a significant number of participants have experience of working in a whole system way. For example, if the planning group for a large event has itself become used to working with the ground rules, they may provide a critical mass of 'self-managers' when they participate in the event itself. A system-wide planning group of, say, 30 people could amount to almost a quarter of the participants and throughout the two or three days of working together they take part in many different groups.

Tricky as it may sometimes be, self-managing behaviour is not something new in human systems. It is the way many communities, families and couples organise their relationships and get things done. Encouraging self-managing behaviour is often about giving people permission to bring into the world of work the ways of being that they naturally use elsewhere.

Not only the hard stuff

From our work over the last four years it seems to us that local systems frequently limit their resourcefulness by concentrating on the hard cases. It is understandable that most energy goes into solving the hardest problems but this often has unintended consequences. For example, while someone needing a lot of support has a very well co-ordinated hospital discharge, another person whose discharge should be unproblematic is left waiting alone in the cold because there is nowhere for their relatives to park when collecting them. Over and over again we have heard from elders that what would make a real difference to their quality of life are things that appear to hard-pressed managers and clinicians as small details – the right sort of footstool, enough pillows, somewhere in the hospital to make tea and toast, 16 wall tiles to be replaced in a shower. These are real problems but they could be solved in all sorts of ways which do not depend on highly specialised teams.

QL [the local shorthand given to a whole system event on quality of life for older people] made me realise that we do not always use our money wisely and well. Older people want simple things that we can't provide. A lot of people heard this at QL and it's a slow process to change things, but I think we're making a start in small ways. (Manager, NHS trust)

Using resourcefulness

In one place, senior managers were particularly concerned about people over 75 and the services they needed. Concentrating on their needs seemed to be the most cost-effective way to operate. They wanted to work with whole system methods and a planning group was formed with people from several local businesses and communities. As they struggled with what they were really trying to achieve and what the system-wide issue was for them, it became clear that their best move was not to limit the age range but to expand it to include younger older people because in that way they were likely to bring more resourcefulness into play.

If a group of people is behaving as an interdependent system, an outsider cannot directly change their pattern of organisation, so what is the role of an outsider like a development agency or consultant? We suggest it is to enable them to uncover for themselves their capacity to adapt and change. We therefore describe our repeated meetings with local partners as 'perturbations'. They often consist of asking questions, particularly questions that do not identify problems or lead to replaying defensive routines. A central purpose of such a perturbation is to cause people to see what they are already doing in a new way, to recognise that there are many ways of seeing things and many possible solutions to problems.

One way of doing this is to design meetings which allow everyone's expertise to be used and to acknowledge that there are many forms of wisdom. This means avoiding formal presentations of expertise or good practice from elsewhere in the hope that they will 'roll out'. If good practice has not already been taken up locally there is a reason for this, and it is unlikely to be simply ignorance. It is more likely that the necessary conditions, the communications network that existed wherever the good practice originated, for example, are not present. The role of the outsider, then, is to enable local people to discover and develop those necessary conditions themselves. When they have done so, they are likely to behave in a way appropriate to their local circumstances. At this stage they may well go and find good practice examples to learn from and adapt. But this follows a choice made inside the local system, and is not *caused by* the external example of good practice.

> ## *Introduce perturbations*
>
> In one borough the local authority had invested a great deal of political will and resources in consulting older residents and drawing up a 'shopping list' of actions to improve services. Many of these had been tackled, reports written on significant progress and articles placed in local papers. Yet there was a feeling among older activists that nothing had changed.
>
> They became interested in working from a whole system perspective and an interagency group began to see patterns linking the ways in which the items on the 'shopping list' were tackled. One pattern was that borough-wide initiatives always seemed to end up with local people saying it would be better to have a neighbourhood focus, so neighbourhood projects were constantly being reinvented instead of incorporated from the start.
>
> Another pattern was that even when it delivered on the 'shopping list', the local authority only got credit when the older people themselves felt actively involved.
>
> In this example the local authority was already committed to consulting local people and trying to do things differently. The whole system 'perturbation' helped them recognise some of the ways they were still 'stuck' despite the hard work.

Whole system working needs more than mere permission from the board level of organisations. It needs an understanding of where possibilities are created in the organisation, who sustains change and who maintains the status quo. If people are to organise themselves to take some course of action, it inevitably means that they will not be doing something else. If the organisation notices and appreciates what was being done before but not the new work, few people will choose to sustain that new work. It needs the active support and encouragement from the top of organisations. People in positions of power have the capacity to stop things happening.

The power to stop

In one place we were working, the medical director of one of the hospitals decided at the last minute that large meetings were a waste of time and withdrew his permission for his clinical staff to take part. The meeting went ahead, and proved useful to most of those who took part, but the absence of a major hospital weakened its impact.

In another place, a city-wide planning group decided to begin their whole system work in two localities, each of which described 'information' as the major issue they wanted to work on, though each had very different ideas about what they meant by this and what they wanted to do. One of the powerful agencies in the planning group felt that it would be wasteful for both these groups to tackle the 'same' issue, and wanted to choose between them. This response was understandable in that they believed that one 'pilot' should be enough and if it worked, its roll-out could be co-ordinated throughout the city. We, on the other hand, expected that very different interventions about 'information' might appropriately evolve in the two very different localities.

We tell these examples not because there is a 'right' way of doing things but because those in positions of power were not in tune with the possibilities and pitfalls of the approach, with the result that a good deal of self-managing activity came to a halt.

Local people, between them, usually know a great deal of what is going on but frequently the knowledge does not flow. Whole system working gives people the opportunity to learn some of the things that do not seem to filter through the usual channels. This is often because it is only the recipients of the information who recognise its importance. In a well-connected group in one London borough, for example, the community liaison nurse was the only person who knew about some respite beds that were underused, despite pressure on the acute hospital nearby. In an inter-agency meeting in another city only one person knew that a home improvement budget was underspent, despite the fact that this was perceived to be the limiting factor in enabling some patients to go home from hospital.

Sometimes it is the new connections and understandings that can arise from whole system working that enable things to happen. Perhaps they would have happened anyway or perhaps it needs special conditions for people to look around and see the possibilities.

Things just happen

❖ A group of Chinese elders discovered how they could lobby to have a bus stop moved to a location that was safer and easier for them to use, and did so successfully.

❖ A voluntary organisation had been seeking funding for an information shop for two years. At a large meeting elders made it clear that a 'one stop shop' was what they really wanted, and the voluntary organisation received funding shortly afterwards.

❖ A group bidding (successfully) for European funding for a major information technology project for small- and medium-size enterprises decided to switch the focus of the bid from railway systems to the organisations that provide services for elders.

❖ A local authority was able 'to hear' that both workers and residents disliked the term 'housing wardens'. The name had unpleasant connotations all round and they decided to change it.

❖ In one borough the laundry service run by the local authority's Leisure Services was under threat of closure because it was not being used to full capacity. During a whole system group talking about services to keep elderly people active in their own homes, the Leisure Services manager heard home helps talk about the problems they had with laundry. He was able to offer the excess capacity to the home help service and prevent the closure.

❖ A social services department decided to transfer its talking-books service to the libraries service – an example of two major local authority departments reaching a new understanding of their own strengths and weaknesses and their clients' preferences, leading to an improved service all round.

Sometimes working in a whole system way gives rise to a climate of improved co-operation and helps people make better use of resources and respond easily to opportunities as they arise. In one borough, two organisations who discovered they were each in the advanced stages of developing a similar project were able to decide to collaborate and thus make better use of resources across the system as a whole. In another, a community care alarm service successfully bid to become part of a substantial European project. The letter of confirmation referred to the 'special relationships' in the local area, which the person who had co-ordinated the bid attributed directly to their involvement in whole system working.

Whole system working requires a real diversity of participants. It enables many people to find renewed energy within themselves and it provides an opportunity to reach out and bring in new people, which in turn increases the chances of using local resourcefulness. The invitation list for one large event, on the well-being of elders, included local artists, a funeral director and the coast-guard. Sometimes working with 'not the usual suspects' leads in unexpected directions.

Bring in new people

❖ The UK head office of an international toy manufacturer, as a local employer, agreed to take part in an event about the winter bed pressures on the local hospital. As a result they became involved with local elders, the education department and others in an intergenerational literacy exchange scheme, which now involves 25 volunteer elders going into local schools. Children are getting access to recycled computers, and the scheme has now received joint funding for a co-ordinator and further expansion.

❖ Another whole system group which continued after a large event were concerned about elderly people in a specific neighbourhood who lived alone and were particularly isolated. Among the participants was a Royal Mail manager along with a nurse, policeman and social services manager. They all felt that nobody had the right information about isolated people. They decided to produce a card with useful telephone numbers for elders to put on their mantelpiece, with space to add the names and numbers of family members or GP or anybody else who might need to be contacted in a hurry. The Royal Mail agreed to distribute this free to all residents. Most significant was the comment of the local authority manager:

Before the whole system event we had never had a conversation with the Royal Mail about anything other than the negotiation of a reduced rate for bulk deliveries.

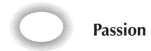 **Passion**

*A living system constantly requires energy
to maintain itself (homeostasis) or to change.*

*If a human system is similar, it too uses energy
to stay the same as well as to change.*

*Whole system working is an approach that releases energy.
Money, time and communication are commonly
recognised as 'fuel'. What is commonly forgotten
as a source of energy is people's passions.*

Organisations may recognise that passion, enthusiasm and energy are important but may expect these qualities from only certain staff – clinicians perhaps or top managers. It is hard to bring creativity to a situation when there is no encouragement to use it. When people are allocated work that is of no particular interest to them or when their enthusiasms are ignored, they may withdraw important parts of their creativity and simply 'do the job'. The loss of energy potential to the organisation can be great. It is worth remembering too the amount of passion and energy that people invest in opposing things.

Our contention is that if the living system metaphor is appropriate, then organisations use up the energy of their staff just to stay the same. If an organisation wants to change the way it operates it has to have energy available to do so. People's passions can be a source of that energy.

When we talk about engaging people's passion we are not suggesting working harder or longer. Instead, we suggest it is energising when people are able to work on something they care about, and when they find that others care too. In practice over the last four years we have found many people who care deeply about what they do and want to 'make a difference' – home helps, doctors, local councillors, managers, neighbours, bus drivers, housing wardens ... the list is long.

Working in a whole system way means putting a great deal of effort into drawing in different people, but we then encourage them to choose to work on things they really care about. Meetings are designed to allow self-selection. This is particularly powerful when people find they are not alone, that others share their passion. And meetings that produce an enormous amount of hard work turn out to be fun too, which in turn raises energy levels even more. We often ask groups to feedback their deliberations in ways which avoid the flipchart or the closely argued report, and never cease to be astonished at the inventiveness that results, and the clarity of the message. One of the outcomes seems to be that people are able to re-engage with long-standing problems.

In formal meetings, certain sorts of evidence are acceptable (aggregate data, analyses, abstractions) and other sorts of evidence are usually perceived to be unacceptable (such as anecdotes, rumours, stories). Those who take part are asked to engage with the analytical side of themselves. This may be appropriate for decision-making meetings but it limits creativity and it excludes some people entirely.

If the meeting has a different purpose – to search out possibilities and new ways of doing things, for instance – then we have learned that it has to be designed to enable people to hear 'inadmissible evidence', to refer to real experiences of how the system works rather than how it thinks it works. These are often expressed as stories and anecdotes. Working in a whole system way means making productive use of these alternative views – Is that how it really happens? Is it always like that? It even seems to be helpful to use the word 'passion'.

The first time we used the word in introducing some work we were asking small groups to do, we were astonished to find that all the reports-back used the word too. Simply using the word passion seemed to have given people permission to engage with the task in a more energetic way than usual. (NB: we refer here to passion *for* something, not against.)

There are straightforward situations where, at least in principle, a clear link can be drawn between cause and effect and people can readily agree on the nature of the problem and the solution. In complex situations, the link between cause and effect is not clear. There is no right answer. There may be agreement about cause without there being a right action to be taken in consequence. There may be no agreement about cause, yet it may be possible to agree about solutions. In these situations, it can be liberating to be asked to contribute without having to reach agreement. It is often quite enough to find others who care passionately about the same issue and want to do something about it. Our experience in practice is that this is particularly so for professionals because acknowledging what others have said is easily translated into accepting responsibility for 'solving it'. If they know they can't do that, the tendency is to find ways of closing down their involvement. Being asked to engage for possibilities rather than solutions feels quite different.

Real stories – the ones you hear and the ones you tell – influence the range of things you can imagine and what you go on to do. Stories can be much more energising than dealing in abstractions.

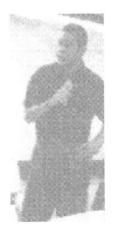

Choosing to act

A chest physician was a member of a planning group enquiring into patients' experiences of being in hospital. She heard a positive story and relayed it back to the group. She had been told about a ward where day-case cataract surgery was carried out. Patients and their relatives had the use of a day-room where they waited and when people came back from surgery they told the waiting patients how well it had gone. As she retold the story, she included the gesture, an energetic double 'thumbs-up', that had accompanied its original telling.

She later commented that this account of mutual support had influenced her thinking about the design of an endoscopy suite that she was planning. Without doubt accounts of mutual support by patients are 'known' in the literature, but it was the energy of the story that influenced the physician's behaviour.

Here and now

A living system operates in the 'here and now'
through many simultaneous interactions and processes.

If a human system is similar, it too operates through
multiple simultaneous processes. It can look messy and
wasteful in contrast to planned, sequential processes.

Whole system working is an approach that gives people
enough time and space to work 'here and now' to establish
shared purpose and meaning and to become aware
of their identity as a system. This enables them to act
at other times and places, whether individually or together,
in ways that naturally support the shared purpose.

Contracting procedures, planning meetings, decision-making committees are some of the formal mechanisms through which organisations carry out their daily tasks. All of them take time and people are always looking for ways of making the most effective use of their time. Frequently, they share a sense of time being wasted, in unproductive meetings or writing reports that are destined to remain unread. In inter-agency working, in particular, the number of meetings to co-ordinate activity can develop into a vicious spiral and the accompanying busyness makes it harder to arrange meetings and essential to keep them as short as possible.

By and large, these formal processes are not designed for exploring possibilities so when that is what an organisation wants to do, it has to adopt working methods which are not sequential like committee-style meetings. This means using time in meetings in ways which encourage richer connections to grow, which in turn allow information to flow in new ways. It also means asking 'what's the bit of work that we have *to do together?'* Our experience is that what has to be done together is to create shared meaning.

A characteristic of whole system meetings is that they are designed to enable all those participating to contribute, often with many conversations occurring in parallel for much of the time. This means designing productive ways of using personal experience, making explicit use of both the past and the future, paying attention to the length of sessions. It also means working in rooms where people are comfortable – natural daylight and good refreshments, for example, and where they can hear what is being said and see what is being recorded. We have learned that detail matters.

We have also learned that one of the most important tasks for facilitators of whole system events is to hold out for enough time. Marvin Weisbord says of the design of 'future search' conferences (see page 128) that at times things seem too slow for some participants and too rushed for others, but it is the fastest way he knows of everybody getting there together.

In committee-style meetings it is often possible to design the agenda in such a way that members need only attend for certain times. Whole system meetings do not work like that: shared meaning needs everyone to contribute and to hear what is contributed. This takes place in real time, the here and now, by which we mean what happens in the moment with whoever is present. When people attend only part of a meeting, they share only part of the experience and this invariably seems pretty meaningless.

What whole system working can do in real time is reveal what people are interested in working on together, and begin to generate the relationships and energy to sustain it. Once these happen, activities can track in many directions through the web of connections. Some of the possibilities which merge will in time be realised through other work processes elsewhere. Perhaps the most significant consequence of sharing meaning in the 'here and now' is that it makes possible a change in climate in which things seem to happen more easily.

Making time

We talked with a small group of senior managers in a borough who were interested in planning a whole system event but were finding great difficulty in contemplating asking people to participate in a meeting which lasted 16 hours over two or three days. They were also doubtful about five half-day planning meetings. A change occurred when one person said, 'I've looked back in my diary at all the meetings I've been to already this year about this issue. If getting all these people to focus on it and work together is really going to make a difference then it'll be time well spent.'

Real-time working

The regional director of a national housing association was so taken by her experience of real-time working in a whole system event that she hired in some round tables, brought together a much wider variety of people from her housing association than usual, and together they wrote the following year's strategic plan in an afternoon.

Patterns of order

Living systems are highly complex, yet stable patterns of order emerge without recourse to external design and control. They emerge from the repeated application of a few simple rules.

If human systems are similar, coherent patterns of order arise from a few principles that guide behaviour. People can choose to change the guiding principles.

Whole system working is an approach that uncovers these self-ordering principles.

There is a fundamental distinction between control and order. Control is usually taken to mean 'checking and directing action, domination, command' with a further meaning of 'restraint'. When somebody gives an order, they are exerting control in this way; but order can also mean 'the condition in which everything is in its proper place, and performs its proper functions' and even 'the fixed arrangement found in the existing constitution of things; a natural, moral or spiritual system in which things proceed according to definite laws'. Order is about pattern, not about detail. Order is about the overall shape of a tree not where a particular leaf or branch is.

Human systems may organise their behaviour around a few rules or guiding principles that are not at the conscious level, and these may change without ever entering consciousness. However, bringing these rules into conscious awareness offers the opportunity to discuss them, investigate their implications, and even attempt to change them.

In the NHS, for example, one of the puzzles is why so much of what happens is unchanging. The underlying nature of the NHS has remained remarkably stable, despite the barrage of attempts at reform and structural change, since 1948. Many behaviours have not changed. This stability could be explained by some powerful guiding principles that shape behaviour and give order to the NHS.

One example is the principle 'can do, should do'. In 1948 this made sense: there were post-war shortages of everything so more was better, far fewer available treatments, and a widespread belief that science brought unalloyed benefits. Fifty years later things are different: we are more wary of technology, the range of medical interventions could swallow the domestic economy, and treatments can be seen as unkind, ineffective, unnecessary, inappropriate and even unethical.

Although appropriate in 1948 at the launch of a universal and comprehensive health service, this principle may now hamper decisions about how to make the best use of the available resources across the whole population. It may hamper the NHS's adaptive capacity. To allow proper reform of the NHS we have to engage directly with these guiding principles, rather than simply changing the organisational structure.

The guiding principles *that people actually use* may reinforce the stated aims and values of the system in which they operate, but they may also undermine them. Uncovering the guiding principles that give order to complex social systems is an intuitive process for which there are no recipes. One method we have used is to get small groups of half a dozen people to engage in the sort of conversations one might have with somebody new to the system who wants to know how it really works, rather than how it says it works. Listening 'between the lines', it may be possible to hear some guiding principles.

Another method we have tried is to ask people to work in pairs and tell each other about an actual experience of, say, going home from hospital. The listener has to try to imagine what the people concerned in the story were really thinking, the inner voices that guided their decisions and behaviour. We have also worked with groups of about 40 people to gather a large pool of statements about the way a system operates, both when it is working well and not so well. People then sort these into three categories:

> **Believe** – the underlying values without which the system would not be the same
>
> **Guide** – the guiding principles or 'rules of thumb', which may be unconscious
>
> **Do** – operational guidelines, which will vary between organisations.

In the example of going home from hospital, an underlying value *(Believe)* was 'patient-centred care'. The operational guideline *(Do)* was 'clear written and verbal information to the person/carer'. The guiding principle *(Guide)* that everyone in the group could agree was found between these two and expressed as 'if in doubt ask the patient.'

> ## Guiding principles
>
> In another place a group of people was gathering stories about older people's experience of a stay in hospital.
>
> For example, one of the disturbing experiences about a stay in hospital is being moved to another ward. It was rarely explained to patients that this might happen as their needs changed and many of the stories were about 'feeling lost'. Mostly, professionals did not tell them until the move was quite certain, leaving little opportunity for the patient to get used to the idea. Professionals seemed to think uncertainty would unsettle the patients. They were particularly reluctant to share this uncertainty because, it emerged, they often felt the moves were unnecessary and arose because of the needs of other people in the hospital. They wished the moves could be avoided.

One of the guiding principles that emerged from this exercise was 'patients are strategists too'. What was meant by this was that patients are often treated as if they are unable to cope, although in most aspects of their lives they do cope. They went on to explore what this might mean in practice, if it were acknowledged as a guiding principle. They agreed that this principle would encourage professionals to explain to patients and their carers not just what should happen, but the range of things that could happen.

An important outcome of this kind of work is that people can see the world differently. One example is the change from trying to achieve order by predicting and controlling detail to recognising and anticipating patterns, and articulating the rules and guiding principles from which they arise. If organisations are seen as mechanical systems with cogs and wheels that need oiling and tend towards disorder, it is the responsibility of those in charge to be continuously fixing and controlling. If, on the other hand, they are understood to be capable of generating their own order – order for free – the role of those in charge is to reveal patterns and engage with guiding principles because this is what enables you to engage at system-wide level.

In summary ... This chapter sets out the principles which characterise whole system working and examples of what this means in practice. We believe that the living system metaphor describes what goes on naturally when communities and families work well, but it is seldom the way organisations choose to work. In essence, the approach is about enabling people to build connections and communication and uncover 'common ground' that they want to work on together. This is easy to say but not easy to do. We use everyday methods of working with large and small groups of people to enable them to share meaning, make connections and explore possibilities for action.

Significant features of these methods include:

* *expertise:* everyone's expertise is used and people participate as individuals, not as representatives

* *diversity:* we work with multiple perspectives as an asset, a resource to the system

* *lay people:* significant numbers of lay people are involved at every stage and their voice helps professionals hang on to a sense of 'the whole'

* *personal experience:* meaning and purpose are hard to get at and often start in discussion of abstractions so we design meetings that get at meaning through stories and personal experience

* *recognise the system:* we work in ways which enable a local system 'to know itself'

* *time:* we build in sufficient time to explore purpose

* *asset-based:* we use working methods that start from capacities and possibilities, rather than deficiencies and trouble-shooting

* *logistics:* we pay attention to detail

* *conversation:* we make constructive use of conversation and dialogue rather than formal speeches and presentations

* *public listening and recording:* this matters when people are trying to share meaning and experience so we pay attention to microphones, acoustics, wall space and so on.

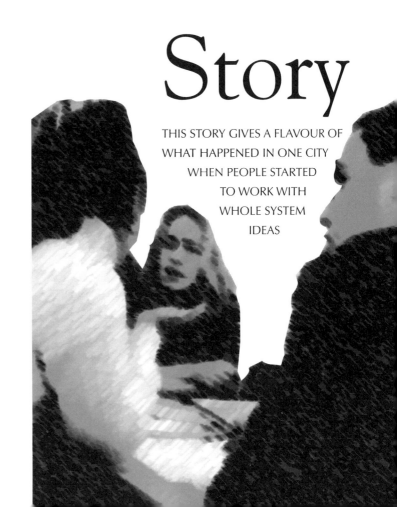

Story

THIS STORY GIVES A FLAVOUR OF
WHAT HAPPENED IN ONE CITY
WHEN PEOPLE STARTED
TO WORK WITH
WHOLE SYSTEM
IDEAS

Conversations and narrative are the currency of human communication. Stories form a bridge between teller and listener and four people listening to the same story will each hear something slightly different. We interpret nuances and fill in gaps in meaning in ways that are based on our own experience of the world. Different perspectives, real experiences and 'conversations for possibilities' are the essence of working whole systems. This is the story of what happened in one city when people started to work with these ideas.

In the early 1990s the Newcastle and North Tyneside Health Authority's strategic objective was to 'rationalise' the hospital service in Newcastle by strengthening community-based services at the same time as closing hospital beds. They realised they had to build closer relations with the City Council, the universities and the many active voluntary agencies in the city. This led to the creation of the Newcastle Health Partnership that brought together the major stakeholders with an interest in improving the health of the city. One senior official said,

> When I heard about the whole system idea I thought 'Yes!' It seems obvious to me that the whole should function as greater than the sum of its parts. The very democratic approach of whole system working is something that promotes the wide involvement needed to ensure that this happens.

A group of people came together in early 1995 to explore the ideas and how they might be used to improve the well-being of older people in the city. They knew that this would depend on a lot of different organisations and on older people themselves, and could imagine that bringing them all together might be productive. So they went to the newly formed Newcastle Health Partnership with a proposal to hold a whole system event. By the final planning meeting in September 1995 more than 35 people and organisations were already involved and on the big day something like 200 people gathered at the Eldon Leisure Centre.

I remember going down the long corridors with a real sense of expectation but also nervousness. There was a tremendous buzz. In the main hall lots of round tables were set up and all sorts of people were milling around wondering what was going to happen.

Participants had all sorts of concerns – would this just be a talking shop, was it worth three days of their time, would their concerns get to the top of the agenda, would the results be anything other than an unrealistic wish list?

To me the essential thing was to suspend disbelief and give the event a chance. I'm glad to say that most people did the same and it began to gather real momentum.

A whole system event is not at all like a normal conference or public consultation. There is no platform, no presentations and no outside experts. Almost a quarter of the participants were older people. They were some of the most enthusiastic, not least because they found themselves sitting around the same tables as senior managers discussing issues that really mattered to them.

Getting chief officers on board is really important. We worked hard at that. The most important thing is that top people are supportive, even if they're not all present.

Local people formed something like 14 or 15 small groups after the event to work on issues they felt particularly strongly about. Some got on quickly with specific work, such as publishing a directory of housing suitable for older people. Some grew in unexpected ways, others floundered.

Hearing stories in a new way

One group started with a concern about the services that older people can expect in their own homes, such as home helps. The group consisted of an older woman and four managers from social services, the health authority and a voluntary organisation.

They had an open remit and an unusual mix of people and in this group the woman concerned had time to share the distress caused by a discharge process that went wrong. Her late husband had been discharged from hospital on a Friday with the wrong appliances and no instructions about what to do in case of difficulty. As a statistic this may not seem remarkable, certainly not an event likely to give rise to significant organisational change. Most people have, after all, heard stories of unsatisfactory hospital discharge. But this group accepted the story as significant in its own right – and they decided to do something about it.

From problems to possibilities

The most natural way to tackle something that has gone wrong is to analyse the problem and set about fixing it. This may be effective when there is a single or simple cause, but not when it's a complex issue involving several different professions and organisations. Why, after all, is the experience of hospital discharge still frequently unsatisfactory after decades of training, policies, guidance, initiatives and strategies?

This small group were beginning to adopt an exploratory approach, perhaps because of their experience of working in different ways during the whole system event. They decided not to analyse the problem of this particular discharge but to use it as a source of energy for change.

The group of five – the four managers and one service user – looked for other people who shared their concern and swiftly brought together a 40-strong group from many parts of the city, including more older people. They shared what they knew about the dozens of initiatives and projects already under way in the city. They realised that each initiative was part of a wider system of hospital discharge, and while each would improve part of the system, there was no guarantee that the system as a whole would work better.

They made an important breakthrough when they changed the language they were using from trying to 'solve a problem' (how to improve discharge) to generating possibilities (how to make going home from hospital a positive experience). This is really significant and more than just a semantic point. Hospital discharge focuses on the institution. It immediately frames the issue as a problem for the hospital – how we discharge someone. It invites organisations to shift the blame – if discharge isn't working it is someone else's fault. 'Going home' turns this on its head. It focuses on the patient. It helps create an understanding of the need for organisations and staff to work together to achieve a desired outcome. It emphasises shared responsibilities to make the system work better.

The group of about 40 people met for half a day at a time, to allow relationships to grow and understanding to be shared. They worked at round tables seating eight – at times with people from similar organisations and at others in mixed groups. They invited extra people along and always included older people and carers. 'No Elders, No Meeting' became a kind of mantra.

What really happens

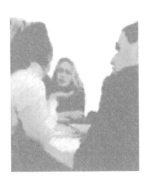

An important early task was to draw a map of the business of going in and out of hospital. This was done by having a facilitator describe an 'archetype', an older person not coping at home due to illness. The group were invited to describe what might happen and the many possibilities were drawn on a wall map. The stories began with the way things are supposed to work but this was such a mixed group of people, who were developing their mutual trust, that they soon started to describe what really happens and how different this looks from different standpoints. This honest sharing of personal experience provided the foundation for everything that followed.

Even the simplest hospital discharge involves a patient, a nurse, a doctor and an administrator in the hospital, transport and a general practitioner. By mapping what actually happens the group 'revealed' the central role played by friends and neighbours as well as family, and the contributions of a whole network of voluntary organisations. They revealed differing expectations of what the GP will initiate in the way of home visits, and what people expect of social workers. They saw the difficulties of co-ordination between hospital pharmacies and the ambulance service. They saw the importance of parking for private cars when collecting patients. They saw the central role that interpreters can play and the number of occasions at which it is the patient who is expected to think ahead and to make links between different bits of the system ... the list goes on and on.

Most significantly the mapping revealed the communication links, delays, interconnections and the many situations in which the honest response is 'well, it depends ...' or 'sometimes what happens is that ...' or 'on a Friday ...'. Even experienced managers were surprised to see the complexity and the mismatch between their individual mental maps of how discharge works and the map they produced together.

A shared list of desired outcomes

At the next meeting, the group was invited to spell out what a good hospital discharge service would look like from each component organisation's point of view. Voluntary organisations, social services, district nurses, hospitals, older people – they wrote their desired outcomes on flipchart paper, cut this into strips each containing one outcome, and grouped them by sticking them on the wall. Each group of outcomes was discussed and sorted by everybody. Many of the desired outcomes were shared by several organisations – such as good communications and patient-centred care. Others came from one group but could be readily agreed by the others – such as acknowledging the needs of carers as well as patients. Others led initially to disagreement – such as the elders' wish to have the final choice of place of discharge. This in turn led to discussions of the real costs of different packages of care and ultimately to a completely new desired outcome – making the best use of the resources available to the system as a whole. It was allowing time for these conversations that provided the basis for shared understanding.

This shared list of desired outcomes formed the basis of a draft strategy document which the group of 40 started to prepare.

A new way of looking at strategy

In a single organisation strategy serves to guide and give coherence to decisions and actions. In a whole system made up of many organisations there is just as much need for strategy but its form has to be different. The mechanism of accountability is different in a complex system – there is no one owner or boss who is responsible for its functioning and to whom people are accountable. Decisions are made in a variety of situations and need to be sensitive to individual circumstances. No one set of rules for hospital discharge could encompass all the possibilities.

What's needed is a new way of thinking about strategy – one that sets out the common principles that guide action throughout the system. The strategic question becomes:

> *What guides our actions if we hold ourselves accountable for the behaviour of the whole system?*

The group of 40 recognised that the common list of outcomes they had produced contained not just desired outcomes but some statements that looked like these guiding principles, and others that were aspirations or values. They separated out three categories:

> **'Believe'** – fundamental values which everybody aspired to and without which the system involved in going home would be something different (for example, 'patient-centred care' and 'make the best use of resources across the system as a whole')
>
> **'Guide'** – principles which are shared across the system and are used to guide the actions, decisions and trade-offs that are made every day (for example, 'if in doubt, ask the patient and their carer' and 'when in difficulty I'll ask for help from, and explain the difficulty to, other parts of the system')
>
> **'Do'** – rules that specify what is to be done and how

Armed with this understanding they worked through the issues to shape a draft strategy on going home from hospital. They tried hard to gain new insights into familiar problems. But this strategy needed more than a group of 40 people if it was to become real.

A whole system event

They got agreement from the chief executives of the organisations most involved to plan a whole system event on going home from hospital. The design for the event was a modification of a method called Real Time Strategic Change. This allows a draft strategy to be tested out with an even wider range of people who contribute to producing the final version.

The event was held in February 1997 and 170 participants came together for two days to work on the question, 'What can we do to make going home from hospital a positive experience for older people and their carers in Newcastle and North Tyneside?'.

It was as though the group had grown once again – from 5 to 40 and now to 170 – but continued to work in the same sorts of ways. People contributed from their personal experience in conversations, often with people they would not normally meet. Those who took part were invited as individuals – not as 'six nominations from the voluntary sector' but as six people personally invited because of what they could contribute. Getting a good mix of people is what matters if new possibilities are to emerge and the group of 40 had worked very hard on the invitation list, as well as the draft strategy.

Over the two days all the participants worked on developing the desired outcomes and the guiding principles and produced a final version of a strategy to make going home from hospital a positive experience. This included a commitment to review the work that different organisations 'Do', in the light of the system's 'Believes' and 'Guides'.

After the event most of the 170 participants were enthusiastic about the experience of working with such a rich mix of people. A video and a workbook were produced to accompany the strategy document and some organisations used these as a basis for action in house to engage even more people. Others, however, chose to involve only a few people within their organisation and thus reduced the potential impact.

One factor that did not work well at this event was the involvement of doctors. They were present but they had not taken part in the group of 40 who developed the draft strategy, although theirs is one necessary perspective on hospital discharge. The group frequently identified doctors as the cause of many of the problems that concerned them. The doctors joined the process too late to contribute to the understanding that had already been reached and this meant that at times during the event their perspective simply could not be heard by others.

Developing strategy in a whole system way involves far more people than usual at an early stage. (More commonly, a few people draft a strategy document and then the organisation puts most effort into consulting widely and cascading the strategy.) And they spend more time together than the usual one-and-a-half-hour committee meetings because of the importance of building communication and relationships. Understandably, some people are reluctant to contribute this time to what sounds like 'just another meeting'. But when a system is not 'aware of itself' and some parts are missing, the tendency to shift the blame is overwhelming.

What difference does it make?

There seem to be three sorts of outcome:

A new climate

The most difficult thing to pin down, yet probably the most powerful, is the emergence of a climate of improved co-operation. People have more connections than they had before. For example, some nine months later when short-term government money was offered to ease the winter beds crisis, a group of people from several agencies involved in the Going Home initiative were able to rapidly put together a successful bid. The resulting partnership was much more than the usual collection of signatures to secure funding.

There is greater respect between agencies. For example, the co-ordinator of a big voluntary organisation was invited to use a health service staff minibus to travel between hospitals. Not only did this make better use of her time, it also increased the number of chance meetings and flows of information.

Elderly people are keen to stay connected. Some of them have worked as paid researchers in an evaluation of hospital discharge.

People are less likely to blame others. For example, a voluntary agency received a complaint from an elderly person about a promised service that failed to arrive. This turned out to be the result of a failure of communication between the hospital and the general practice but rather than shift the blame, the person from the voluntary organisation contacted the others and worked out a way of ensuring it would not happen again.

Pop-ups

Some things happen very easily as a result of new connections and understanding. These just 'pop up' – they could have happened anyway but were helped along by a whole system perspective. After the Going Home event, staff from the community care alarm service met with the housing department and the community health trust and agreed to become the communication link for the out-of-hours district nursing service. This in turn led to better co-ordination between all three services.

New initiatives

Some completely new things happen. A housing department and a community health trust have set up a new nurse-led intermediate care unit in a sheltered housing scheme. Two hospitals have redesigned their discharge groups to bring in a much wider membership, including voluntary agencies. All the organisations involved in the Going Home event have publicly endorsed the strategy, and most have reviewed their own policies and guidance.

In summary ... In this chapter the 'going home' story gives a flavour of what it's like to work from a whole system perspective. It is a method of working which is neither 'top-down' nor 'bottom-up' but makes use of the wisdom and enthusiasm of many different people who have a shared concern 'to make a difference'.

Transferability

DESPITE THEIR DIFFERENCES, BOTH PRIVATE AND PUBLIC SECTOR
FACE SIMILAR ORGANISATIONAL CHALLENGES
IN A WORLD OF INTERCONNECTED NETWORKS.
WHOLE SYSTEM WORKING IS WIDELY APPLICABLE

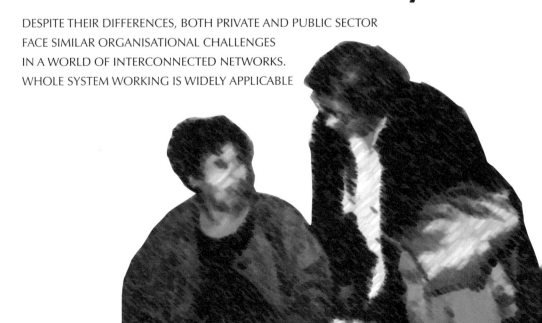

The examples in this book come from the public sector but the whole system approach we describe has much wider applicability. The context, the players and the purpose of the public sector may be very different from the private sector, yet the organisational challenges they face are similar. Commerce and industry, as much as the NHS, grapple with dense networks of interconnections. The potential for disruption that stems from the inability of computers to recognise the year '2000' is a startling demonstration of the web of interdependencies that nowadays connect organisations. A failure in a computer in one organisation will have multiple but largely unforeseeable impacts elsewhere.

In less dramatic ways organisational commentators have long been stressing the need for linking, synergy, networks, partnership and integration in order to create 'learning organisations', which make full use of their human talents. These concepts are about relationships between relatively autonomous units, not the more traditional view of integration and co-ordination based on direct management and vertical integration. General Motors, for example, once owned the plant and directly employed the labour for every stage of car production, from mining iron ore to selling cars. Over time they realised that their special competence was car manufacture. They did not need to manage or own the whole business of the car production system but, to ensure that it operated as a 'value-added-chain', they would need to pay attention to the connections between the various parts.

Having a systems perspective means that we have to give as much attention to the fit between parts as we do to the design of the parts. But a cluster of organisations does not constitute a system. Donald Schon has said that often organisations are 'memorials to old problems', institutional residues which reflect the historical process through which problems have been tackled. In a rapidly changing world, organisations which see themselves as living, ongoing communities may be the most adaptable. Decisions need to be based on fitness for purpose, rather than historical precedent or institutional power or habit. And this means considering the possibility of co-evolving behaviour in which all the players have to contemplate changing and becoming something new. The company Prêt-a-Manger is an example here. A group of architects began to specialise in designing premises for the modern generation of sandwich shops. They worked in partnership with catering companies, each bringing their respective expertise and co-ordinating their efforts. The products were very different in style and ethos from the older fast food outlets. Finally, they realised that they knew more about this sort of business than the catering companies so they changed from being architects to form the chain of shops known as Prêt-a-Manger.

Richard Normann uses the word 'offering' to describe what it is that service industries deliver. These offerings are often intangible and ownership is not transferred. Production and consumption frequently happen in the same moment and place and the service user takes part directly in the production. Service organisations have traditionally adopted a 'relieving strategy' – bring us your problem and we will fix it – but this too is being challenged. If we see the client as an active and integral part of the service, then both provider and client add value. This is co-production and leads to a view of the organisation's purpose as enabling clients to meet their needs, rather than relieving them of their needs.

The quality of any service is determined by the face-to-face work between an individual provider and the client. The higher the status of the provider, the greater their degree of personal discretion in the performance of their work. But, wherever the service is provided, it is the personal interaction that is a large part of what is created. We learned this in discussion with the corporate strategy group of one of the High Street banks. It is clear to many senior managers in businesses such as these, which are complex and widely dispersed, that most of the organisation's capacity for innovation is found at the frontline. Yet there is a tension between the centre's need for control and accountability and their need for the periphery to act autonomously and creatively. If these organisations can think of themselves as a living system, then it is possible to think about strategy and change in new ways. Many of the practical methods we have been working with address the same issues – the need to build relationships which release the energy and potential within the system. McMaster describes this management task as creating the conditions to support 'conversations for possibility'.

The context of our work is the public sector and, specifically, a rapidly changing NHS. When we began we were interested in so-called intractable problems, the ones which prove remarkably difficult to tackle, despite the hard work and good intentions of many people. If problems prove to be intractable then, by definition, old ways of working have proved to be inadequate. Our hypothesis was that the problems we were interested in would be interpreted differently by different stakeholders and the difficulties in reconciling these would in turn contribute to their intractability. This meant we were inevitably drawn to another well-recognised problem: boundaries – between services, between agencies, between sectors, between professions, between government departments. As the public sector becomes increasingly deregulated, boundaries between agencies multiply. Since boundaries are frequently the site of failures of communication, understanding, respect and co-operation it is not hard to see that the problem, and possibly the solution, lies in cross-boundary working.

We struggled with questions like:

Can one person or agency ever have the whole picture in a system made up of many related parts?

Do problems remain intractable because 'ordinary' ways of working simply do not address them?

Do quick fixes fail because they invariably address symptoms and not causes?

Does any intervention in a system have knock-on effects elsewhere, and are they unexpected?

Could the overall performance of a complex system be improved simply by attention to the parts?

For us thinking about London's health services illustrated the issues raised by questions like these. Research, training and education, and service provision all pull in different directions. Interdependencies cannot be mapped and there are major weaknesses in information. There is no way of harmonising regulations and procedures. There is no overall system of governance. The net effect is that although each element may be organised in a way which appears effective, the system as a whole performs badly and its capacity to learn new ways of working is limited. The paradox is that while collaboration and partnership are seen as the answer and hard-working people put great effort into getting their bit right, the whole seldom seems to add up to the strength of the parts.

In summary ... We suggest that the whole system approach has wide applicability and that organisations which see themselves as living, ongoing communities may be the most adaptable in a rapidly changing world.

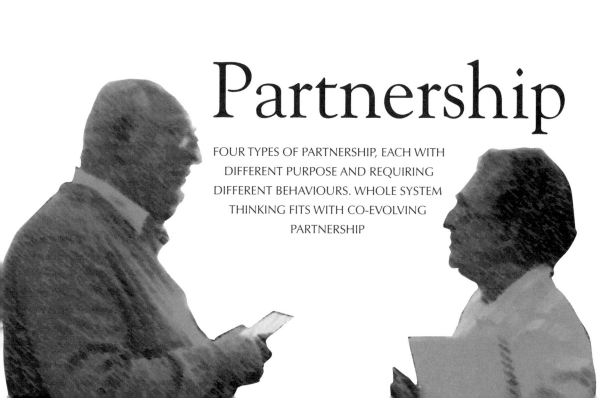

Partnership

FOUR TYPES OF PARTNERSHIP, EACH WITH
DIFFERENT PURPOSE AND REQUIRING
DIFFERENT BEHAVIOURS. WHOLE SYSTEM
THINKING FITS WITH CO-EVOLVING
PARTNERSHIP

We are emerging from a period when competition was promoted as *the* effective means of achieving social outcomes. Now partnership is the political imperative – between private and public sectors, across public sectors, between professionals and lay people, and with citizens generally. Many people welcome the shift in policy. They share the Government's aspirations for partnership working, yet it sometimes feels like the triumph of hope over experience.

We have found it liberating to recognise that there are several different sorts of partnership behaviour (Fig.4). What seems to matter most is that there is clarity about the purpose of a partnership. We distinguish between competition, co-operation, co-ordination, and co-evolution. Each requires different behaviour to achieve its ends and when these behaviours and purposes get muddled up then the frustration with partnership grows. These forms of partnership are not a hierarchy but an attempt to describe different circumstances and the behaviours appropriate to each.

The horizontal axis in Fig. 4 represents the different types of goals being sought. To the right, people and organisations are pursuing individual goals. To the left, the goals are collective.

The vertical axis represents the extent to which the purpose and the behaviour needed to achieve it can be known in advance, plotted as predictability. In the lower half, objectives are recognisable and the way to achieve them is understood. The future is predictable if you understand the present and the way things have worked in the past. In the upper half, on the other hand, only broad aims can be recognised. The future can be anticipated but not predicted in detail. Achieving the goal will depend on triggering changes in other partners.

The distinctions between the four corners are not watertight. Real partnerships include elements from several at any one time, and are likely to move between them over the course of time. Nevertheless, the distinctions can be useful in recognising the behaviours that are likely to be appropriate in different circumstances.

Fig. 4 **Partnership behaviour**

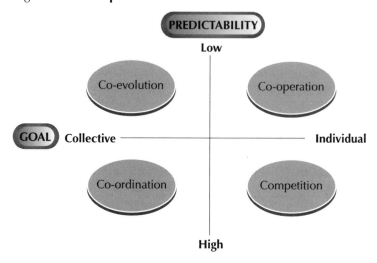

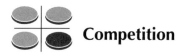 **Competition**

Competition may seem an odd place to begin but it is not a solitary behaviour and it is a powerful tactic for change. In the bottom right corner of the diagram the goal is individual (either personal or organisational) and clear and everyone understands the ways to achieve it. Competition can be a powerful stimulus for improving creativity and the efficiency of individual parts of a system, which is often exactly what is needed.

■ *Example*

Hospitals compete for junior clinical staff in order to fulfil their service contracts. When staff are scarce, competition is likely to make each hospital ask itself what it can do to make it the kind of place junior staff want to work in.

Competition should be the simplest form of 'partnership' behaviour to bring about and the easiest to sustain, as it requires no agreement (or indeed direct communication) between competitors and there are no uncertainties about what to do.

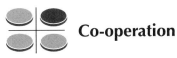 **Co-operation**

Even when each player is motivated by self-interest, there are situations when co-operation is a better strategy than competition. Co-operation arises when the goal is individual but the partners see their future as linked. They act to influence the behaviour of other members over time because, instead of the win/lose of competition, there is the possibility of win-win.

■ *Example*

Hospitals co-operate to run junior doctor rotas. By offering an employment package to which they all contribute they can attract the staff to fulfil their individual service contracts.

The good news about co-operating partnerships is that they do not need the time and effort required to reach a collective goal. They do need a structure that penalises those who act competitively and rewards those who co-operate. And they need a sense that their futures are linked. One-off activity is not enough because co-operation may only emerge as the best strategy over time.

If you are in a position to influence the environment in which the partners are operating and you want to encourage co-operation you would want to:

- promote trust and communication
- enlarge the 'shadow of the future'. The most serious barrier to the evolution of co-operation in organisational life is the lack of continuity of relationships – from the past and into the future. If people move frequently from job to job, there is no opportunity to have the iterative interactions with other players that are required to trigger co-operation. And if people and organisations do not expect to have to keep working together (or even if they can see a date for the end of the relationship), the incentives to co-operate fall off rapidly. Shaping the game to promote co-operation therefore requires creating stability in relationships, avoiding reorganisations, building expectations of length of stay in jobs and so on
- design a structure which penalises individuals who act competitively, while rewarding co-operators and long-term behaviour. Living within one's budget while cost-shifting would no longer be acceptable behaviour
- teach the players about the benefits and strategies for co-operation – particularly by encouraging them to make their decision rules consistent and transparent
- allow players to interact mainly with others who also use co-operative strategies. This allows co-operation to begin to flourish and then spread to others.

Among *organisations*, co-operation may be one of the most underused forms of partnership. Its surprising advantage is that it doesn't need a collective goal. Among *individuals* it is probably the mechanism by which a lot of business gets done – 'you scratch my back and I'll scratch yours'.

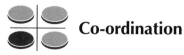 **Co-ordination**

More akin to the everyday usage of the term partnership is co-ordination, which we place in the bottom left corner of Fig. 4. Solutions are knowable from past patterns, as with competition, but the difference is that the goal is collective.

Co-ordinating partnerships come together with the intention of delivering pre-set, common objectives. There is confidence that the objectives are the right ones and this is based on past experience of what works. The driving force in this environment may be a desire to reduce duplication, to add value by pooling resources or to fit the parts together better. This is the jigsaw model where, as long as everyone shares the same picture, they can in time see how all their separate pieces fit together.

■ Example

When hospitals share a common goal of training junior staff with colleges of education, local authorities and health authorities, they form a partnership (education consortium). Each knows the part they have to play to achieve the goal. They still operate independently – they may even be competitors on other issues – but for the shared goal of training junior staff they operate by co-ordinating their contributions.

Project management is a tried and tested form of behaviour here. Everyone has to do their own part of the work but in a sequence or manner which allows the whole project to be completed. There are clear and joint objectives and these are known as the project begins. There are timetables and targets, and individual roles are usually specified in both qualitative and quantitative terms. This is the environment in which the master plan can work, particularly when outputs can be clearly specified. In house building, for example, contracting processes are well rehearsed. Regulations are clear. Value-for-money frameworks are set. At a technical level it is relatively easy because people know how to behave as contractors and suppliers.

Co-ordinating partnerships are frequently limited to issues that do not challenge the individual goals of the organisations concerned. They are most successful in important areas which are nonetheless not core business of the partner organisations (e.g. interpreting services for health professionals and minority ethnic communities, transport schemes for housebound people). This form of partnership rarely 'infects' the core business of the partners, who continue to pursue their individual goals. Their activities are more like worthy organisational hobbies and often do not survive beyond a 'project' period.

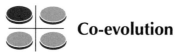 **Co-evolution**

Sometimes partnership is needed to generate new possibilities and new ways of working. We place this type of partnership in the top left corner of Fig. 4. The goal here is shared but less clearly defined than the pre-set objectives of co-ordination and there is no certainty of what works.

In this environment we use the term co-evolving partnership to describe behaviour in which the partners are committed to co-design something together for a shared purpose. This is about lifting the game to a new level of operation. It is not about past patterns that are known to work or about co-ordinating known good practice. It is about working together into the future, which is not yet knowable. The timeframe is long and the collective goal much less clearly defined than the objectives of co-ordination. To follow through the junior hospital staff example:

■ *Example*

If the shared goal were to become not just the training of present day clinical staff but the future workforce of the entire health care sector, then the nature of the partnership would have to change. Many different perspectives would have to be drawn in. The timeframe would be longer; the future uncertain; and the first task would be to create conditions where long-term productive relationships can thrive.

Partnership in this 'co-evolving' sense is a vehicle for engaging with seemingly intractable problems and we think this is where whole system working has much to offer. We also think it's got lots going for it when people are curious about how-do-we-do-things-differently-around-here and start looking for partnerships for possibilities.

This typology offers a way of thinking about the purpose of partnership and the different behaviours which are appropriate under different conditions. The nature of the collective goal is one of the critical links between the quadrants. We don't need it for competition. We don't need it for co-operation to succeed. We don't always get it right in co-ordination – we think we've got it then it turns out to be something else, often to do with money. For co-evolving partnership to thrive sufficient people need time to explore purpose and understand why they are building relationships. The whole system approach fits in this top-left corner. We suggest that this is where many of the long-standing and complex issues around social exclusion and regeneration can be located. They are likely to be influenced by the actions of many different people and organisations. There is likely to be broad agreement about aims but no precise objectives and the levels of complexity are likely to be such that no clear path can be mapped out to achieving them. We think that whole system working has a lot to offer both as practical methods and as theory that guides action.

In summary ... This chapter offers a way of thinking about the purpose of partnership and different sorts of partnership behaviour which achieve different ends. The example on the following pages further illustrates this concept.

Booksellers and partnership behaviours

None of us is a bookseller but when we look into that world we recognise a range of behaviours which fit the partnership typology:

- Bookshops compete for customers. Until recently they did not compete on the basis of price but on things like opening hours, location, audio-tapes and so on. As the big chains started to cut prices, small booksellers have had to find other ways of adding value for their customers. Some have branched out into selling coffee, stationery, children's play corners, internet access.

- Sometimes booksellers both compete and co-operate. Second-hand booksellers seem to be particularly good at co-operative behaviour. In several market towns in Britain when you visit a bookshop, you will be given a map showing all the bookshops in town. We don't know how this began but the bookshops seem to have decided they have more to gain than lose and the assumption is that if one co-operates the others will too. Often these bookshops carry much the same stock but there is a degree of specialisation – one has more children's books, another more art books (and the latter will also direct you to the artists' supplies shop). Suppose the town's tourist office wanted to encourage this co-operative behaviour, they might decide to produce a map and thus change the pay-off structure for booksellers. Those who co-operate by distributing the map and referring customers are rewarded by being included. The sanction against those who 'defect' is removal from the list. The tourist office would be acting here as the 'rule-maker' intent on promoting co-operative behaviour among the town's shopkeepers and starting with those who are already inclined to do so. This win-win behaviour may lead to other co-operation which is not visible to the customer, such as sharing warehousing arrangements.

- Book-selling is the major economic activity in the town of Hay-on-Wye in Herefordshire. Booksellers, and many other interested parties, share a common purpose which goes beyond selling books to attracting potential buyers to the town. In recent years they have successfully acted together to co-ordinate the Hay-on-Wye Book Festival. Marquees are erected, B&B offers are encouraged, international advertising commissioned, special promotions featured, famous authors invited, prizes awarded and lots of visitors welcomed to the town.

- An example of a co-evolving partnership is the internet-based bookshop, Amazon, and its customers. Amazon has the explicit intention of creating a community of readers – when you buy a book you become a member of Amazon. If you are interested in deserts, Amazon can tell you what others with similar tastes are currently reading. It can make links beyond books, for example with the suppliers of outdoor equipment. As a bookseller Amazon has to compete with other bookshops on price, range, convenience, reliability, speed of delivery and so on. Technology has made it easy for Amazon and its customers to interact at any time of the day or night. Through home-based computers they have succeeded in making themselves more accessible to many people than neighbourhood bookshops. They have changed the environment in which local shops compete. Of course, many people still want to browse, to meet others, to be tempted by an unknown title rather than place a pre-decided order. But booksellers may be influenced to think differently about how they lay out their shops and how they behave with customers. Meanwhile, Amazon has made use of the interactive capacity of its technology to encourage its customers to write their own book reviews, which are made available to other readers. Now you can tap into a global network to find out what people think about the book you are contemplating reading or add your bit to this creative community. Will this virtual community develop and begin to organise itself in other ways? Will Amazon evolve into a different sort of organisation that influences trends in publishing in new ways? No one is certain what will happen next.

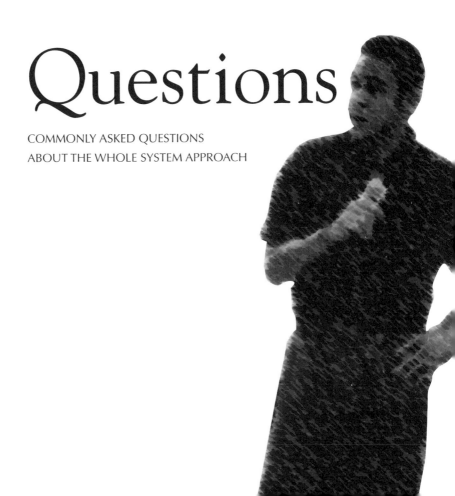

Questions

COMMONLY ASKED QUESTIONS
ABOUT THE WHOLE SYSTEM APPROACH

? Aren't we working as a system already?

Almost certainly, yes. Most people operate as a part of several systems, and these change over time. At a formal level organisations churn away all the time with systems of accountability, planning, performance management and so on. You can think of this as a mechanical system with appropriate cogs and wheels operating as a well-oiled machine. You almost certainly operate as part of human systems as well which don't feel like a machine, more like a constantly adapting, organic entity. That's what this book is about – organisations as complex, adaptive living systems.

? If I don't like the way things are working what do I do?

It depends. If you see your team or organisation as part of a well-oiled machine then when it doesn't work as you would like, you expect it needs redesigning or reorganising – better information systems, perhaps, or monitoring mechanisms or new planning structures.

If you see things operating as a living system then you recognise many interconnected parts that make up 'a whole' which is capable of adapting and evolving. Living systems of this sort organise themselves anyway, all the time. So, if you don't like the way the system is organising itself, you need to encourage it to behave in a different way. That means you have to intervene at a system-wide level because you know that concentrating on the parts alone won't deliver the overall change you are seeking. First, you need to find a way of 'making the system aware of itself' and then of 'giving the system access to itself'. This in turn will generate new connections and new information flows and these are what create possibilities for change.

[?] Is this instead of traditional change methods?

No. It is not a substitute for other work processes, all of which have their place. It is an additional tool. We think it can be a means of engaging with long-standing, policy-resistant problems, the ones which never seem to go away despite the efforts of highly motivated people 'on the ground'.

[?] How do you engage people with power?

Whole system working is not an approach you can 'sell' if people are not curious. Our experience is that a lot of senior people are looking for new ways of operating and it feels more like tapping into the 'zeitgeist' than having to convince them. They seem to recognise that there is a lot going for this way of working because:

- people are tired of 'quick fix' change
- financially constrained services have to find effective ways of working across boundaries to make better impact
- there is disillusion with short-term, project-led funding
- however instinctively, there is a growing awareness of systems thinking and complexity
- effective partnership working is now an imperative, not an 'organisational hobby'
- involving lay people in developing services is a requirement
- for good or ill, policy makers are interested in systems thinking.

[?] Do we need to create a new system if we want to work differently?

No, you don't need new parts but you almost certainly need new connections. If you want to work differently, you start with what you've got – the existing gene pool – but you have to think about how people can reconnect differently. You need to 'make the system aware of itself'. If a network of people has a shared purpose they have an identity, but they may not be consciously aware of it. When people recognise themselves as an interconnected system, opportunities increase and different questions have legitimacy – like how does my behaviour affect the behaviour of the system as a whole?

? So what happens as a result?

We have learned to anticipate lots of energy and enthusiasm, new connections, new working relationships, shared experience, a rich network of contacts, a climate of improved co-operation and less likelihood of blame-shifting. These in turn create the possibilities for new ways of working. You can't predict what will happen locally because everywhere is different but examples include:

- speeding up some things that are already in the pipeline (e.g. funding for a one-stop information shop)
- modifying existing work (e.g. altering an EU information technology project to focus on housing needs of older people)
- pop-ups, things which could have happened anyway but seem to happen very easily as a result of new connections and understanding (e.g. two agencies discovering they were developing similar schemes and deciding to collaborate)
- new initiatives (e.g. older people working with social services to monitor the quality of services in residential homes)
- creative opportunism (e.g. having the relationships and information in place to bid successfully and at short notice to become a pilot site for a government programme).

? How does this way of working fit with formal structures?

It fits by offering you another strategy. It gives you a way of operating in the top-left corner of the partnership typology on page 100. Organisations need both formal structures and partnerships for possibilities so it's not either/or.

Throughout joint working arrangements there are many formal structures in operation – contracting procedures allow you to compete and to co-ordinate, performance targets and joint planning mechanisms allow you to co-ordinate and so on. In time, some of the possibilities which emerge through co-evolving behaviour will be realised through formal structures elsewhere.

It also fits through people. The same people who gain information and shared understanding from operating in 'possibilities mode' bring this to bear on their other work in more formal settings.

? Do we need a lead agency?

Having a lead agency is usually a means of holding one agency accountable, and that is not appropriate here. The whole system approach is good at developing a sense of joint responsibility. This is one characteristic of a system 'being aware of itself', so it's not appropriate to create another hierarchy. You probably do need an organisation to act as 'host' mainly for administrative purposes, but that is not the same as accountability.

The other thing to remember is that this way of thinking is not simply about inter-agency work – the notion of 'the whole' and 'the parts' and how they connect has as much relevance for a single organisation and human enterprises of all sorts.

? What do you mean by 'an approach'?

It is a combination of new ideas and practical methods of working. We think it is the strength of this combination that creates the conditions that enable people to re-engage with long-standing problems.

It's not a toolkit – more like a tune in the back of your head. If you are interested in the principles of whole system working (see pages 23–78), you'll be keeping your eyes open for ways you're already operating that could be adapted.

? Does change always involve large numbers of people?

Change in organisations always involves large numbers of people, whether they are invited to take part or not. Usually, the many people who must take part in implementing a strategy are involved after the initial design process, which is left to the responsibility of a few.

The approach we describe recognises the potential contribution of people with many different perspectives. The question then becomes, how do you work constructively with the great diversity in a complex system? If this requires working with large numbers of people, we are confident that there are effective methods for doing so. Some of these bring large numbers of people to work together. Others involve large numbers of people but do not necessarily bring them together.

Our view is that it is purpose, passion and meaning which build coherence in complex human systems – in which case the more people involved, the better.

? What does a whole system event cost?

There are two sorts of cost – those which are borne by the local system and those which are paid for 'up front':

*   costs borne by the system:
    – participants' time to take part in a planning process
    – participants' time to take part in a whole system event
    – administration to build up a participants' list, issue invitations and co-ordinate activities after an event

*   costs paid for up front:
    – facilitators to design and lead the planning process and the event. These costs usually vary from 10–25 days' work depending on the degree of sustainability you are aiming for and the follow-through you want to invest in
    – domestic costs such as meeting rooms, conference venue, printing, food and so on. These too will vary depending on what local agencies provide 'in kind' and the numbers of people involved.

? So what's the distinctive benefit of a whole system event?

If your aim is to change the system's behaviour then adopting this approach will get a great many people connected and their attention focused on a shared concern. The real investment is in the use of people's time. One hundred and twenty local people working together over two days is about the equivalent of a whole year's work for one person. You might, for example, decide to employ a liaison worker to make connections and build an understanding of the system and its possibilities and to share this with local organisations. Or for comparable cost you might prefer to get 120 well-connected local people, and the possibility of changing the system's behaviour. Value for money will depend on your purpose.

? Can you really trust the system?

Again, it depends. If you believe that human systems organise themselves whether or not they are subject to formal control, then the answer is, 'Yes, you can trust the system *to organise itself*'. Our experience is that if the right mix of people is brought together and meetings are designed which enable them to work constructively, then we can trust their judgement. And lots more people are involved in creating possibilities than usual. (What you can't do, of course, is trust the system *to do what you want*.)

? When is it worth taking this approach?

When you recognise that you are looking for new ways of working and that more-of-the-same just won't produce new solutions, no matter how hard people try.

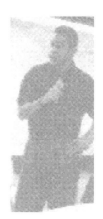

? How do you make sure participants are representative?

You need people from 'every neck of the woods' but this way of working is not about finding representatives. Our experience is that the methods which are successful are designed to allow everyone to participate as an individual, not as a representative. Participative behaviour is about taking personal responsibility, whereas representative behaviour is about expressing views clearly and handing over responsibility for action to others.

? Is this just better consultation?

No. Consultation is about asking for and providing opinions and advice (e.g. responding to plans made by others, seeking feedback on existing services, assessing what the community wants). Consultation serves other purposes too (e.g. informing the public, gaining legitimacy for decisions, or permitting dissent to be heard). There are lots of ways of doing it – focus groups, citizens' juries, questionnaires, public enquiry and so on.

The whole system approach we describe has a different purpose. It is about all the parts of a system co-producing something together for a shared purpose. Lay people or service users or the public are not separate but an integral part of the system. Consultation in the usual sense is just not an option.

? Is it 'the event' that really matters?

Yes and no. The prominence of an event is both attractive and problematic. Yes, it matters. Any large group meeting engages a lot of people and is very public. It can be a stimulating and productive way of working together, but this alone won't change the system's behaviour. In our view a large group conference only becomes a whole system event (WSE) under certain conditions and then there is the possibility of the system choosing to change the way it operates. The WSE is part of beginning to work differently.

? What's the legitimacy for working this way?

Organisations need both formal structures and mechanisms to generate possibilities. This approach does not replace other working methods. Its legitimacy arises from making explicit the shared purpose of a wider range of people than are usually involved, from finding out what people care enough about to work on together.

? How does accountability operate?

Being accountable outside formal hierarchies is based on holding oneself accountable *for* something, for behaving in ways that support the purpose of the system. It is not about being accountable *to* someone.

[?] Is this community development 1990s style?

Again, it depends how you see things. Community development can be seen as a way of contributing effectively to organisations by enabling local people to add their voice, to supply a missing part of the jigsaw. In this sense whole system working is different in that it involves *all* participants (local citizens, board members, middle managers, operators) in co-creating the future.

Community development can also be seen as enabling a local community to take action. Whole system working is similar to this sense of community development but it includes organisations as well as communities. It's not bottom-up but neither is it top-down – it is about all levels of power working together.

We are struck by the notion that ideas take a good twenty years to take off. If this is so then a lot of people who are now in positions of formal authority were around in the 1960s and 1970s and interested in community development. Whole system working is not the same but it does have overlaps – like an upward spiral rather than going round in circles.

[?] What does real time work mean?

Real time is what happens here and now, not a preamble or planning but what happens in the moment. In whole system working the bit of the work that takes place in real time is about creating shared meaning and relationships. Once these are in place, then the detail of actioning the work can take place anywhere. What whole system working can do in real time is to bring to the surface what people are willing to collaborate on, to produce together – the so-called common ground – and to generate the relationships, energy and information flows which can sustain it.

This way of working contrasts with much committee work, which serves a different purpose. A committee takes stock of what has happened since the last meeting and agrees what needs to be done before the next one. The committee's principal task in the here and now is to make decisions in an open and accountable way that is minuted and leaves an audit trail.

? Is this about creating consensus?

No. It's not about reaching a broad consensus on what action to take. If everybody has to agree what to do often nobody ends up particularly excited about anything. It's not about looking for the right answer or about ironing out differences. It's more about bringing into the open lots of different perspectives out of which possibilities may emerge. It's about being *clear* about purpose and meaning. Sometimes it's enough to simply bring these to the surface. When people find there is more shared understanding than they realised, then that too leads to unexpected actions.

? What about sustainability?

Our experience is that local systems can find their own solutions to their long-standing concerns. They're not likely to be new inventions. They may be new to some agencies but are almost certainly known somewhere – it's the process of uncovering, rather than importing or inventing solutions, that generates the possibility of change which is not only locally appropriate but sustainable.

Events

DESIGNS FOR LARGE GROUP MEETINGS AND WHEN THEY
CAN BE USED AS WHOLE SYSTEM EVENTS

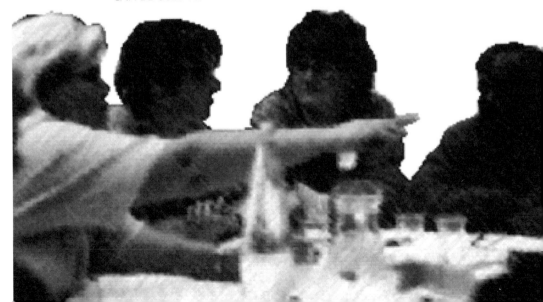

In this chapter we describe some of the principles underlying the design for large group meetings, which are not just scaled-up small groups. We also describe the context in which large group meetings can be used as whole system events – that is to say as events that contribute to sustainable change in the ongoing life of a system.

Large Group Interventions is the name given to meetings designed specifically to allow large numbers of people to work together at the same time in the same room. They may last several hours or several days. They can be entirely successful one-off conferences. Participants may number hundreds or a few dozen and they are responsible for contributing what they know and for doing the work. There are usually no outside speakers.

Sometimes meetings involving large numbers are planned as though they were scaled-up versions of small groups though they are known to exhibit different dynamics. Most people have experience of working in small groups. There is an extensive literature about the design, dynamics and facilitation of small groups. Good experiences of taking part in large group meetings are less common, for several reasons:

- *voice* – it is difficult to ensure that all participants contribute, are able to hear the reaction of others, and are recognised for their contribution
- *dialogue* – it is difficult to create the possibilities of dialogue that goes beyond the restating of the opinions people brought with them
- *mood and feeling* – the mood of a large group is contagious and can swing rapidly, at worst becoming a mob.

Over the last 50 years a range of designs for large group interventions has emerged through the interplay of social psychology, psychoanalysis and systems theory. These designs enable all to have a voice; provide time to nurture relationships and establish genuine communication; and benefit from the potentially mood-enhancing capacity of working together with the same aims. These designs are now sufficiently familiar that they are no longer 'special', and are being increasingly taken into mainstream business meetings.

If you think of commissioning a large group intervention you will want to find a practitioner who will plan and design the intervention with you, and then facilitate it. Each large group intervention has its own purpose and detailed design that tackles the issues of voice, dialogue, mood and energy. To suit your particular circumstances the practitioner may suggest a unique design, or modifications to one of the well-tried designs described in the literature. (To find out more see page 126 and the annotated bibliography.)

By far the best way to get a sense of what large group interventions feel like is to attend one either as a participant or as a steward. The next best way is to watch a video.

Just as with small group processes, people attending a large group intervention may experience a wide range of feelings. These depend in part on the design, preparation and attention to detail, and in part on what hopes and fears they bring to the meeting. Most participants find large group interventions enjoyable, participatory and energising. But there are potential pitfalls:

- when participants have a shared history of opposition and conflict, the use of an inappropriate method can exacerbate the feelings
- when participants have no shared history or future, or when the issue is one they do not feel passionate about, these methods may feel deeply frustrating
- when these interventions are well-designed, they can provide the fastest way for all the people in the room to share understanding and move to action. However, some participants find parts of the events too slow, while others find parts too rushed

- most participants find it easy to adjust to the behaviour and working methods of other participants, but some find these infuriating
- people who attend for less than the full duration always find it a waste of time.

Large group interventions have limitations. They involve large numbers of people for significant lengths of time. They require careful planning, attention to detail of the logistics and experienced facilitators. They should not be used when you can achieve your purpose in easier or more familiar ways. They are not an effective way of, for example, consulting the public or implementing a planned reorganisation.

When certain conditions are met large group interventions can be *Whole System Events* and can alter a system's behaviour. In our view a whole system event is part of the ongoing life of an adaptive human system. It is not a one-off event. The theories underlying the design of large group interventions are not the same as the theory derived from the living system metaphor.

If your aim is to change the system's behaviour then the attraction of working simultaneously with large numbers of local people is that their time and attention are focused on a shared concern in a very public and energising way. But holding a whole system event is really no more than a broadening out of a way of working to include a greater number of people in the building of networks, sharing of purpose and exploration of possibilities. It is not unusual after an event to find members of the local team who have planned and organised it saying 'as far as I am concerned the planning process was more important than the event itself'. And so it should be for them.

Whole system events may be designed especially to meet the needs of a particular situation. Or the design may start from one of the well-tried designs for a large group intervention that is then modified appropriately. One essential aspect of whole system events compared with large group interventions is that sufficient numbers of the people involved must recognise that their futures are linked, that they are part of an ongoing interdependent system. While whole system events can be described as large group interventions, not all large group interventions can be described as whole system events.

Five established designs

● System mapping

Systems mapping enables participants to recognise the complexity of a system of which they are a part, and understand better how it works.

We begin with an 'archetype' – a description of a situation whose essentials repeat themselves again and again, though not identically, as in a stereotype. For example, a woman in her late 70s has a 'turn' at 10 pm one evening when she falls over and seems a little confused. This is a situation that is recognised as immediately familiar to people with experience of older people. Participants describe how this situation might develop and this is mapped in public, on the wall. If participants have time and trust each other they will eventually begin to describe how things *really* happen rather than how they are supposed to happen.

Rationale

We initially developed systems mapping as a 'diagnostic' method that would allow us better to understand a local system. Participants immediately recognised it as an intervention in its own right. We believe its success lies in the way it engages with people's own experience; enables conversation in the group; and leads most participants to a genuinely enhanced understanding of their experience by hearing other perspectives.

What it feels like

Participants get a real buzz out of sharing and learning together in a mixed group. It raises energy and it can be difficult to stop.

Limitations

The method only works if the archetype is recognisable and if there is a good range of perspectives present. The map itself has meaning only for those who have taken part in the conversations that accompany its construction.

What happens as a result

Participants develop a much richer understanding of the system of which they are a part and a recognition of its complexity. They often confront their own assumptions about the way the system actually works – recognising the ways in which actions taken by one person or organisation frequently have unexpected consequences elsewhere in the system. Other things can happen as well as the development of new understanding. Participants build their own network of relationships. Sometimes things 'pop up' – the new understanding leads immediately to action. Systems mapping is particularly useful early on for a group wanting to take the whole system approach.

● Open space technology

'Open space technology' enables groups of 5–500 participants to manage the content of their meeting, which may last anything from three hours to three days. They have the opportunity to put on the agenda items they want to discuss, and then choose the discussions they want to take part in. Reports from each discussion group are stuck to the wall for all to read, and may be copied and distributed later.

Rationale

'Open space' trusts that people usually have the capacity to organise their own work if they are provided with a structure. 'Open space' is probably quite close to the minimum structure necessary for this self-management. Harrison Owen, its designer, says that 'Open space runs on passion bounded by responsibility' – responsibility for taking the theme as the boundary for the discussions, for participating and, when appropriate, for making sure that something gets done afterwards.

What it feels like

'Open space' can feel wonderfully liberating as a way of working. Its alias, 'the all-day coffee break' sums up the experience. It can also feel pretty terrible – particularly if the organisers are trying to control the outcome; if participants are not passionate about the theme; or if there is a history of conflict that has not been acknowledged. But managing one's own work to the extent of leaving an official meeting when somebody is droning on about something that doesn't interest you is not to be missed.

Limitations

Once the 'open space' begins, the organisers have no control about what discussions take place. It is a method absolutely to be avoided when the 'right answer' is already known or when people believe it is the responsibility of a small group of experts to come up with the 'right answer'.

Preparation

One of the great attractions of 'open space' as a large group intervention is the fact that it often needs very little preparation, and can be arranged at short notice. If it is used as a whole system event, the planning takes much more time and effort to ensure that the issue is carefully refined and that a diverse mix of participants from all parts of the system turns up on the day.

What happens as a result

The emphasis on self-management ensures that most people get a lot out of meeting in this way, and that useful discussions take place. Whether anything happens afterwards depends on the issue and the participants. If the aim is discussion, the discussion takes place. If the aim is the production of a report, this can be produced during the meeting. If the aim is action, this may continue afterwards.

• 'Future search' conference

'Future search' is a tightly choreographed design that provides the opportunity for participants to spend two days creating their shared future together. They begin by building up a shared understanding of their past. They move on to honest conversations about how things are now, giving groups and organisations the opportunity to tell others what they are proud of and sorry about, and for the others to endorse those 'prouds' and 'sorries' they feel are important to bear in mind for the future. This brings participants to the point where they are ready to imagine a shared future that is grounded in the realities of the past and present but which is aspirational. Groups present their imagined futures back to the whole conference in imaginative ways, and the shared themes from these futures are brought together in public to form the 'common ground'. In the final session participants select whichever 'common ground' theme they feel most passionately about and work together to plan what they might do after the conference to take it forward.

Rationale

'Future search' builds on earlier designs and a thorough understanding of large group dynamics. It relies on the wisdom and resourcefulness of the participants both to contribute their own experience as the content of the event and to manage their own small group discussions.

What it feels like

Walking into the room at the beginning of a 'future search' is quite a shock for most participants. The room is full of round tables, each with eight seats. There is no platform, no expert speakers. Within 20 minutes everybody is on their feet, writing on large sheets of paper on the wall and contributing their experience of the past.

The core work of the conference is carried out at the round tables in conversations, each of which has a clear theme and purpose. At the end of each conversation these are fed back to the whole conference in a variety of ways using roving microphones. Most participants find

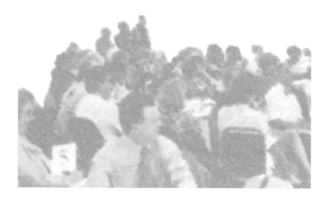

the conversation groups satisfying as there is a chance for everybody to contribute, and feedback to the large group is remarkably easy. There are peaks and troughs of energy over the two days but most participants leave feeling energised and part of a wider whole.

Limitations

Provided that participants do have a shared past and the possibility of a shared future this is a robust design that most people find really satisfying and enjoyable. If participants just come together for a conference it can be deeply unsatisfying.

Preparation

'Future search', like all the other large group designs, requires meticulous attention to the detailed logistics. What happens during the conference depends on who the participants are, which in turn depends on the issue that has been chosen and the care with which they have been recruited.

What happens as a result

The impact of a 'future search' conference does not occur as a result of a written conference report but as a result of changes in behaviour among the participants that arise from a new way of seeing things. If there are people who are key to making things happen as a result, you have to find a way of making sure that they are there at the conference – for the whole duration. The groups who plan to take things forward afterwards often need some support and nurturing, particularly as their members go back into organisations that have other priorities.

● Real-time strategic change

'Real-time strategic change' meetings allow a wide range of participants to spend three days contributing to the development of strategy. A typical meeting begins with a welcome from the 'top people' and an invitation to all those present to contribute to the organisation's strategy. Experts, from outside and inside the organisation and including customers, give presentations that describe the environment of the organisation and some predictions about likely trends. Groups within the organisation have honest discussions about which of their contributions to the organisation they are proud of or sorry about, and share these with the conference as a whole. They identify what other groups in the organisation could do that would enable them to do their job better, and make requests directly to them.

Before the event a strategy team have prepared a 'straw-man' strategy document. All participants discuss the document in groups and share their comments and suggestions with the whole conference. The strategy team then have the task of re-writing the strategy document overnight and circulating a new version for the final day. They present back to participants the changes they have made, and explain why they have not made other suggested changes. Participants conclude by agreeing how they will implement the strategy.

Rationale

'Real-time strategic change' is based on the premise that everybody in an organisation is capable of contributing to its strategy, and that people are more likely to implement something they have had a hand in creating.

What it feels like

This is not what people expect when they are asked to contribute to a strategy document. Working in groups of eight at round tables allows good conversations. It is a lively design with peaks and troughs of energy, and is generally very successful in building understanding and commitment.

Limitations

It requires considerable openness from the strategic level of the organisation. Although the strategy team never let go of responsibility for the document, if they choose to ignore what participants have said this is exposed in public. Probably the major limitation is the nature of the written strategy document, which may have an analytical form that is difficult for participants to engage with.

Preparation

The logistics and participant list are, as always, of crucial importance. A key element is the process of preparing the 'straw-man' strategy document. If this is produced using the same sort of processes as are used in the conference – conversation groups and many different perspectives – much of the most important work has been done beforehand, and the conference serves to check it out with a wider constituency.

What happens as a result

This can be a quick way of producing well-informed strategy. More significant is that, by putting time and effort into the early stages, the strategy is more likely to be implemented.

● Appreciative inquiry

We include 'appreciative inquiry' in this chapter because it can be used to engage large numbers of people. It is not a large group intervention but its originator, David Cooperrider, often uses it along with large group techniques.

'Appreciative inquiry' replaces the traditional problem-solving cycle (Diagnose, Plan, Intervene and Review) with the possibility-finding cycle (Discovery, Dream, Dialogue, Destiny).

In the discovery phase people share stories of exceptional accomplishments, discuss the core life-giving factors of their organisations, and deliberate upon the aspects of their organisation's history that they most value and want to bring to the future.

The dream phase challenges the status quo by envisioning a more positive and vital future – not out of thin air but grounded in examples from the positive past. It begins by valuing what has been found in the interviews by feeding them back in a report or meeting. This is assisted by constructing 'provocative propositions' – statements that bridge the best of 'what is' with your own speculation or intuition of 'what might be'.

The design phase involves creating the organisational forms that reflect and support the dream, and the final phase is an invitation to co-create the future – the opportunity to build the appreciative eye into the way the system works.

Rationale

Appreciative inquiry recognises a problem with problem-solving – that focusing awareness on the deficit between the actual and the desired supplies negative images and negative dialogue.

'What we ask determines what we find. What we find determines how we talk. How we talk determines how we imagine together. How we imagine together determines what we achieve.' (David Cooperrider)

What it feels like

Taking part in interviews about positive experiences is often very liberating. To hear, or to tell, what it is that has made a particular situation – for example a city, an organisation, a team – positive and life-giving can enable people to re-connect with hope and possibility and give them energy.

Limitations

If people have not had the opportunity to express their anger and frustration, asking them to focus on the positive can seem like just another insult.

Preparation

The choice of topic, crafting of the interview questions and training and support of interviewers is key to success.

In summary ... In this chapter we discuss the design of large group interventions and the conditions under which they can be used as whole system events. While whole system events can be described as large group interventions, not all large group interventions can be described as whole system events.

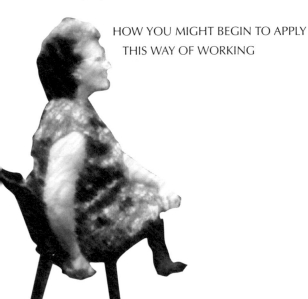
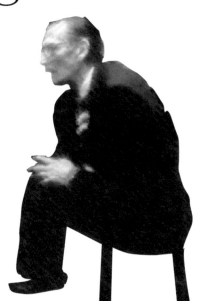

Where to begin?

HOW YOU MIGHT BEGIN TO APPLY
THIS WAY OF WORKING

Whole system working is not a 'toolkit' but we sometimes describe it as akin to 'mood music', like a tune in the back of your head. Once the mood music is playing, it is a matter of finding opportunities of amplifying what is already there. If you find resonances in what you have read so far then you will be alert to ways you are currently operating which could be adapted. It is about doing everyday things differently, as well as doing different things. Thinking about how you could design ordinary meetings in new ways perhaps – who is invited? Are they all at the same organisational level? How can you introduce more perspectives? Or about designing a staff induction process that includes a conversation to explore purpose with someone from another part of the organisation. Or about designing a programme of inter-agency shadowing and secondment. Or about inter-professional training which involves lay people and so on.

If things are not going as you would like, rather than trying to control them in the usual ways, can you find out what purpose is being served by the present behaviour? Can you find some way in which the people involved can get clear about what their purposes really are? When somebody new joins the organisation, listen to what people say when they explain the way things *really* get done around here.

Whole system working is not a substitute for other work processes, but it has a lot going for it if your purpose is to generate new possibilities and new ways of working, the co-evolving behaviour described on page 104. When people start to see things from a whole system perspective, they find a variety of ways to take it into their own situation.

Doing everyday things differently: self-managing

An experienced manager, Ms P, was in charge of the consultation exercise on the local authority's community care plans. The authority had good relations with the voluntary sector and about 80 people were expected to attend a one-day meeting. Some months earlier Ms P had taken part in a whole system event and become really interested in the process. For the consultation exercise she decided that, instead of using facilitators to run the small discussion group sessions, she would ask participants to work on the self-managing principles of the whole system approach. She was quite fearful about how this might be received by her colleagues.

After the formal presentation of the plans, she asked participants to sort themselves into groups of eight and to make sure they were as mixed as possible. The groups were asked to work in a circle. She gave very clear guidance on the small group task and how to self-manage it.

Her aim in all of this was to use the opportunity of the day to get people engaged in ways that could become mutually productive, not just reacting to the local authority. She was pleased with the outcome, especially the way people felt included and able to contribute. But when she told this story some weeks later she emphasised how hard it had been to hold her nerve about no facilitators.

Doing everyday things differently: perspectives

Community health trusts provide an enormous range of community-based health services. They employ both generalists (such as district nurses) and specialists (such as paediatric teams and physiotherapists). They work with general practice, with social services, with local hospitals. Sometimes the relations between community trusts and general practice are strained. General practice is currently being reorganised into primary care groups (PCG).

One of the directors of a community trust, Ms G, wanted to improve relations between trust staff and local general practices. She knew of whole system thinking and began by forming a mixed group of 25–30 trust staff who reflected the many different professionals employed by the trust. She designed a meeting which invited them to explore their own role in creating the present situation. This illustrated the limits of their knowledge about their 'opposite numbers' in general practice. The participants expressed a desire to know more. She felt the meeting had managed to avoid the 'usual response' of shifting the blame.

She designed a second meeting with the aim of allowing this large group to experience a conversation between 'the sides', general practice and the community trust. Three people from the trust talked with three people from general practice using a 'fish bowl' technique, which allows the large group to sit in a circle around the six people and listen to their conversation. Ms G took care to have several perspectives within this conversation so as well as frontline staff she included a manager, a doctor member and a lay member of the board. They were invited to talk about an area of joint concern, not about a right or wrong way of doing things.

Doing everyday things differently: possibilities

The social work department of a hospital was being merged with local authority-based social workers. A middle manager from social services, Ms C, was asked to convene a meeting to take forward the new arrangements. She anticipated about 30–40 people would attend a two-hour meeting. She too had taken part in whole system events and decided to try to get at some of the possibilities of the new arrangements. She borrowed round tables, asked the social workers to work in mixed groups of six to eight people and then to feed back their deliberations to the whole group. Everyone participated, the discussions were lively but the meeting was completely hijacked by the hospital social workers. It emerged that this was the first opportunity they had had to talk together about the reorganisation.

Their resentment about the way the change was being handled dominated the meeting. They were not ready to think about possibilities. Ms C was not only disappointed but shaken. The meeting had gone in unintended directions and she felt responsible for unleashing strong feelings.

When she told this story she reported feeling as though she'd got her fingers burnt but then gradually discovered that people were still talking about that meeting months later and how useful they had found it.

Doing everyday things differently: language

A group of middle managers from several agencies were talking about their aspirations for the New Deal for Communities initiative. They all had experience of several regeneration programmes. They were excited by the possibility of making a sustainable difference, this time. The notion of 'sustainability' was greeted with nods and agreement, not surprising in a well-intentioned group of managers with quite a lot in common although they work for different agencies. Had the group been more mixed, the word might not have had so much meaning.

We described how in one city facing a similar challenge, after a while they began to use the phrase 'will it still look good for my grandchildren?' This became the test for sustainable investment decisions.

One of the managers in the group had used the phrase 'something that lasts'. The group became very animated by the possibility of engaging local people in a question like, 'What do we do that makes things last around here?'.

As the conversation continued it was not clear whether they were excited about asking people what it is that they (in the statutory agencies) do which helps things last or whether the 'we' in the question included local residents. It is important to really press this point as it is key to who is in this system and who is out, and so who is responsible for participating and taking action. This was a first conversation with a horizontal mix of people, different agencies at the same level. They cannot assume this form of wording will grab other people's interest. They will have to hold more conversations and in more mixed company in which they too listen hard for what excites people.

We describe whole system working as 'an approach' because we want to indicate its influence in shaping every aspect of our work. It is an approach which aims to deal with 'the whole' and not 'the parts'. It uses the living system metaphor and operates itself in ways which are non-linear. So we have set out the characteristics of the approach (which we can think of as 'the parts') as a constellation, or a wheel (see Fig.3, page 25). In this wheel order and sequence may vary and lots of processes take place at the same time. The wheel is a device for hanging on to a sense of 'the whole', while at any moment giving attention to one aspect.

Our contention is that it is this understanding of 'the whole' that offers a genuinely new way of working. What we are looking for are ways in which *a system recognises it has to seek solutions at a system-wide level, not in its parts.* For this to happen, attention has to be given to three essentials – language, people and design.

Language

Most problems most of the time are dealt with entirely appropriately by individual professionals or departments or businesses. They are not concerns for a wider system. It is therefore really important to be clear that there is a system issue, something that the system wants to tackle, not just one agency or one profession. You are looking for a system-wide issue for which you do not already know the answer. The way the issue is described enables people to recognise whether it matters to them or not, and whether they can imagine doing something about it. Language is critical.

For example, simply restating the current description of a problem may do little more than increase frustration with seemingly intractable issues, and the prospect of more fruitless meetings. New solutions are unlikely just because the problem is stated in a new forum. Old conflicts are likely to be reproduced as the people taking part struggle once more to have their version of the answer adopted. What would improve hospital discharge/the treatment of young offenders/house-letting policies? – these are more like statements than real questions.

The way we ask questions often reflects beliefs about 'whose problem' it is, and 'whose responsibility' it is to solve.

Whose problem ...

If there are long waits in casualty departments is this a problem for the department? Are the solutions about reorganising that department or are they to do with clinical practice in other parts of the hospital, in general practice, the availability of community nurses, the local authority's community care policy, or all of the above?

If your car can't be repaired because a part is not available, is it the garage's problem? Or is it something to do with the distribution system that involves garages, distributors and manufacturers?

In complex interdependent systems there is no simple connection between cause and effect. Problems may be experienced in locations a long way away, in both time and place, from their causes. Peter Senge shows us that the way we ask questions about the problem may perpetuate investment in 'fixes that fail' through tackling symptoms rather than fundamental issues. If you see every problem as a nail, then you keep on reinventing hammers. And 'shifting the blame' is common behaviour in complex systems. Working to identifying a system-wide issue, something that only the system can address, is an important part of the process of seeing things differently.

Finding the language to describe the issue is something that can only be done locally; it cannot happen outside the system if it is to have meaning. We have experience of the wording of this sort of question being imported from one city to another by an external consultant. This can feel hopelessly happy/clappy to local people struggling with problems. The process of describing the issue and crafting the question has to take place locally and in ways that are consistent with the overall approach, the characteristics described in the chapter on Principles. In other words, the language must take into account multiple perspectives, participation, meaning and so on.

Finding the right language is part of attracting people and spreading a sense of ownership. In whole system working the way we describe the issue must invite people to participate in agenda-building, not just reacting to pre-formed problems. If people participate in creating the agenda, then there is no need 'to sell' the solution to them subsequently. We believe this is an important part of uncovering sustainable solutions.

If we form questions around deficits, we may exclude groups whose involvement is critical to new solutions, and so perpetuate shifting the blame. We attended one multiple stakeholder conference where the issue was 'what to do about youth crime?' There were many different people present but no young offenders, nor any other young people. The conference did not produce new energy to make a difference and young people continued to be seen as the problem.

This contrasts with a different approach where the original concern was teenage truancy from school but the system-wide question became: 'How do we make this a place where our young people can thrive?' The latter question mobilised a very different 'system' which extended far beyond the formal education and policing networks. And re-articulating the problem in ways which tap into people's passion for something can release different forms of energy.

Finding the system question, the language to describe the problem, can illuminate the boundaries of the system in new ways. This in turn is part of opening up new connections and new possibilities.

People

Whole system working is about new connections, new information flows and new possibilities. For this to happen you need sufficient mixes of people. Once you have a sense of a system-wide issue, the boundaries become clearer but you still have to identify individuals. Some of these people will probably be obvious but we suggest you also look for 'not just the usual suspects'. You are looking for people who are well connected, in different networks, both formal and informal, in organisations and communities. You are looking for people who want to do something with you, not just to offer or seek advice. In our experience, they must be mixed in a number of ways:

- different levels within an organisation and across organisations, chief executives and front-line staff; planners and operators; clients and managers. All are necessary and customers, clients, service users and citizens are essential because their perspective is especially useful in helping the system recognise how it really works rather than how it thinks it works

- people who know how to connect and are interested in doing things differently, as well as those with formal power

- significant proportion of people with continuing relationships. It is tempting to think that if sufficient representatives of organisations are brought together for two days, then somehow 'the system is in the room'. But if there is no commitment to future action, then what you have is a sample of each kind, an ark, not a system. This shared future is essential for sustainable change in a system's behaviour.

Design

This is about choosing working methods which allow people with many different perspectives to work together productively to uncover new possibilities for action. These methods can be designed for use in large or small meetings. They are not a substitute for planning processes or formal committee-style meetings which usually have different purposes. Instead, they are about participative ways of working that provide time for conversations that allow people to get clear about their purpose.

There are parallels with adult learning techniques. There are critical points in our lives when we absorb lots of data, as children do in language acquisition. As we grow older we retain the capacity to absorb new things but information learned passively rarely affects practice. Hence the limitation of lectures (and books). Mostly, we learn through an active process of interpretation in which we make sense of new material in the light of our experiences of operating in the world and how we believe things work. To reflect this insight, adult learning methods are designed to help people make connections between new propositions and their existing beliefs, feelings and experience. This will be familiar to many people under the banner of experiential learning or action learning. If you are seeking to work with the ideas in this book, you may find yourself revisiting these methods.

You will be looking for a way of spending time together that allows you to explore a range of possibilities before focusing on a particular course of action. You will be looking for ways that allow you all to participate and contribute stories from your personal experience. If the group gets to be more than about 12, this conversational way of working requires particular care and attention to the meeting design.

We are particularly aware of this when we are asked to meet a new group of, say, 20–40 people to introduce them to the whole system approach. We always ask for the room to be set out with 5f-diameter round tables at which six-to-eight people can sit in mixed groups and engage in conversations together for at least some of the time. It is difficult for those hosting the meeting to see that this sort of detail is important, but people behave in quite different ways from when the same topics are addressed in a single large group around the board table.

In our experience methods which work successfully are designed to allow:

- everyone to participate as an individual, not a representative
- everyone to work from experience
- conversation as the unit of currency, so attention must be given to the detail of acoustics, tables and so on
- trust, that local solutions will emerge
- enough time.

In summary … This chapter considers ways you might

begin 'doing everyday things differently' when you start to see things from a whole system perspective. We go on to suggest that genuinely new ways of working come when a system recognises that it has to seek solutions at a system-wide level, not in its parts. For this to happen you must pay attention to three essentials: language, people, design.

Where we began

HOW OUR INTEREST IN WHOLE SYSTEM THINKING BEGAN AND THE ACTION
RESEARCH PROGRAMME ON WHICH THE PRACTICE IN THIS BOOK IS BASED

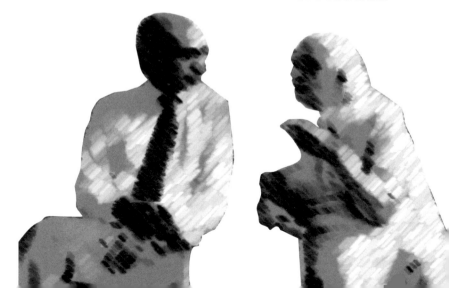

Here we describe how our interest in whole system thinking began and the significance of our base in the King's Fund, a charitable foundation charged with promoting the health and health care of Londoners. We then summarise the action research programme on which the experiences in this book are based, the Urban Health Partnership.

Our interest in looking for new ways of working came from two directions (at least): the debate within the King's Fund about the role of a charitable foundation at the end of the 20th century and a growing dissatisfaction with change initiatives which fail to make an impact on mainstream services.

What's the role of a modern foundation?

Like every organisation, the King's Fund has to pay attention regularly to its prime purpose. This has been interpreted in many ways over the years and has been the source of much lively discussion in recent times, not least because 1997 marked the Fund's Centenary, and serious anniversaries are always good for reflection. But also the environment in which we operate is rapidly changing and deregulation of the public sector is having a significant impact on the behaviour and priorities of organisations in the health and social care world.

The King's Fund is in the business of change. Whether by giving grants, publishing research findings or influencing policy-makers, we have to believe that what we do will make some difference to the services which have an impact on the health of the people who use them. As a foundation, we could argue that our agenda must be in the interests of the whole system of care, rather than the individual parts. In the internal market, we could no longer assume that what is good for a single institution is good for the NHS and what is good for the NHS is good for its users (this may always have been a doubtful proposition and is now patently so). So ideas about who we work with, the nature of the contract with our collaborators, and the distinctive role of a foundation were worth seeking. Several aspects particularly interested us:

- *Boundaries:* boundaries and transitions have multiplied as the public sector becomes increasingly fragmented and these boundaries are frequently the site of failures of communication and respect. The challenge to inter-agency and inter-sectoral working becomes greater than ever and, with the 'joined-up' thinking of a new administration, a great deal now rides on the notion of partnership. Foundations are well-placed to broker the kind of cross-boundary relationships that do not take place spontaneously between enterprises of very different size, culture, power and accountability.

- *Timescale:* in a world of short-termism one of the distinctive contributions of a foundation is steadfastness and patience, the ability to stick with issues for a long time. To do this a foundation has to have its own agenda and be prepared to take risks. Often this means building sustained working relationships around a fairly stable group of issues. This in turn means a commitment to evaluation which is intended to be participative and formative, rather than producing end-point judgements. Outcomes may not be predictable, and may not be reached, but there is a commitment to understand why.

- *Participation:* what does participation with communities mean for a foundation? When resources are scarce, local agencies sometimes have difficulty in seeing beyond the grant money. What constitutes 'good enough' involvement of local stakeholders for a foundation to commit to a longer-term relationship?

- *Grant-making:* the sums of money that foundations have to give as grants are tiny compared with investment in the public sector. At the same time the spirit of philanthropy is thriving and family foundations are springing up all over, not least in the USA and Germany. These are seen as a conduit for private resources to flow into the public sector and there is an interesting debate going on about effectiveness and the alternatives of 'engaged grant-making' or 'disconnected donors'. Simply giving money away is no longer seen as having sufficient impact. The added value of a foundation seems to come from technical assistance backed up with 'soft' money. This lays emphasis on an action/research framework and an obligation to support learning from development initiatives.

- *New methodologies:* in a rapidly changing world we know that 'more of the same' is not enough. Foundations like the King's Fund are in exactly the right place to encourage new methodologies and to experiment with different ways of working. And perhaps one of the most interesting places for the Fund to focus on in the next decade is urban life. What makes a well-functioning city work? Why do some NHS initiatives work erratically or not at all in cities? Could commitment to the health of Londoners be seen in terms of urban initiatives be they about public spaces, transport, health services, employment or environmental sustainability?

Complexity and transferability

We have long experience of primary health care development in cities. Primary health care, that is health care outside hospitals, is one of the main building-blocks of the NHS and its future, yet there is a long-standing concern with 'the problem' of primary care in inner cities. In an attempt to understand this we often try to explain it in terms of some deficiency in one or other part of the system – something wrong with inner city GPs/with inner city populations/ with the quality of management and so on.

We began to think about it in other ways – perhaps it is not that the parts are 'wrong' but that the way services work in cities is different. Perhaps some of the intractable problems in the area of primary health care stem from the irreducible complexity of the system. Much of this complexity results from the relationships between organisations and the range of professionals within them. If this is so, then long-standing problems will not be resolved by trying to effect change through demonstration projects in selected places. To learn from experimentation and then transfer that learning to other settings is difficult. It requires effective teachers, unambiguous experimental results and comparable organisational context. An isolated project is unlikely to achieve this combination and, anyway, learning needs to be effected by the people engaged in the system: it is they, and not the transient project worker or evaluator, who need to understand the system in which they work, especially if they want it to change.

For us one of the driving forces in seeking a new development approach was a sense of growing dissatisfaction with the project approach to change. The belief that the pilot leads the way, the learning is distilled and the best practice rolls out was no longer credible. Good practice *can* be extremely helpful as evidence and in making things real for us, but our experience is that transfer does not readily happen. Instead, all too often what happens is a failure either to learn the lessons of earlier investment or to deliver desired outcomes. The project looks like a fairly harmless and temporary organisational device but is in fact a paradigm – a whole way of thinking about the world which can distort the priorities of the host organisation and play havoc with the delicate balance of relationships and managerial accountabilities.

In 1994 we were in the position of developing a new action research programme which became the Urban Health Partnership. When the Partnership was being formed we consulted widely among charitable trusts, community groups, general practitioners and networks of health professionals and managers. Three clear messages emerged:

- not innovations – what was wanted was help with the long-standing problems of inner city primary care
- not projects – while the need for investment is great, it is hard to bring about lasting change with short-term project money which has to be bid for on a competitive basis
- not more of the same – try to find a way of doing things differently.

The Urban Health Partnership Initiative

The background

Originally founded in 1994 as the London Health Partnership (LHP), the Urban Health Partnership was a five-year development programme focusing on community-based health services. It was set up as an alliance of charitable foundations, government and private sector chaired by Liam Strong, then chief executive of Sears plc, and managed by the King's Fund, one of the contributing foundations.

The Partnership was formed at a time when the Government was investing heavily in projects aimed at 'getting the basics right' in primary care through the London Initiative Zone. The programme grew out of the King's Fund experience of supporting demonstration projects in primary health care in London.

The brief

The LHP brief was 'to do things differently and to add value to the many good projects which foundations can choose to support at any time and to the Government's current investment in improving the basics of primary care'. This was to be a 'learning fund' to find new ways of using relatively small amounts of development money to try to have an impact on mainstream investments. It was recognised there would be no 'quick fixes'. We were charged with developing an innovative programme. We interpreted 'innovation' not as a search for novelty but, in industrial terms, as the stage which follows invention and prototype and focuses on bringing a design into production.

The purpose

- To find new ways of using development monies to bring about lasting change
- To add value to efforts to improve primary health care in cities, particularly services for older people.

The focus

The focus of the programme was improving services for older people because they:

- tend to have multiple needs and experience of chronic ill health
- tend to make use of a wide range of services
- often live alone and are relatively poor, like many city dwellers
- have a lifetime's experience, are often resourceful and want to contribute to the communities in which they live.

The focus comes from our early consultation with health and social care agencies. This revealed no shortage of ideas but a passionate concern that competitive bidding for short-term project funding was deflecting people from what they thought was more important work – the intractable issues – such as mental health services, care for children in poor families, care at 3 am and care for vulnerable older people.

The geographical focus was London, but from the outset it was clear that the issues facing London's health services were mirrored in other cities. A parallel programme was started in Newcastle and North Tyneside and in Liverpool. The work was with health agencies and their local partners in housing, local government, transport, police, the independent sector and local people. An Urban Primary Care Network was formed and met regularly at the King's Fund to exchange ideas and information. The programme was evaluated by a team of locally based researchers led by Professor J. Popay of the Public Health Research and Resource Centre, University of Salford.

Phase one

We consulted widely with health and social care agencies as the LHP was being formed. Once the focus had been decided, our next step was to consult elderly Londoners to hear their *personal experiences* and try to turn these into opportunities for improving services. We set up London-wide meetings and we ran local workshops in four districts to learn about the *barriers to change*.

Personal experiences

The concerns raised by older people in these initial meetings have been repeated over and over again as the LHP programme has developed. There is such consistency that these concerns must be seen as lessons of importance not because of their novelty but because of their familiarity. They include: safety and security, access to services, affordable and accessible transport, independence in the home, admission and discharge from hospital, information about services.

These are concrete problems but beneath them lies the desire for independence, community and affiliation implying a broad socio-economic and even spiritual view of health. It is not difficult to see how these concerns interconnect. People who plan and deliver services and those who use them recognise that responses must be multi-agency, that users must be involved, that professionals must collaborate – these are not contentious issues. What we found to be lacking was effective processes and mechanisms for making them happen.

Barriers to change

We worked in four districts at different levels – neighbourhood, general practice population, operational management, and at policy level. Each workshop brought together between 15 and 30 people already working to provide services for older people in their patch. The system of care around older people involves many agencies and individuals extending way beyond the statutory services. It was this complexity we wanted to understand.

For example, in one district we mapped the progress of a hypothetical elderly person with a minor stroke being taken to the Accident and Emergency Department at 10pm. It gradually became clear that people in one part of 'the system of care' around admission to hospital knew little about the reality elsewhere, and that what appeared to be a solution in one place merely shifted the burden elsewhere, often in ways which were unintended and counterproductive.

In another place there was widespread agreement about the importance of mobility and transport, whether by mini-cab or ambulance or an arm-to-lean-on, and yet transport services were seen to be quite unconnected to other local services.

We learned that if the right people are brought together they can gain a much clearer understanding of the 'big picture'. And that the people who use services bring crucial insights into the way the system actually works, rather than the way it thinks it works. We concluded that anything which helps the health and social care system to understand itself as a whole is likely to lead to better judgements about using resources to bring about lasting change.

Phase two

Phase two is the subject matter of this book and a series of working papers on Whole Systems Thinking, details of which appear on page 166.

Appendix: London Health Partnership Consultative Board and Operational Group

Board

Chairman : Liam Strong, Chief Executive, WorldCom International

Dr Jo Ivy Boufford, Dean, Robert F Wagner Graduate School of Public Service, New York

Robin Broadley, Baring Foundation (to April 1997)

Neslyn Watson Druee, Special Trustees for St Thomas' Hospital

Rev. Dr Charles Elliot, Dean Trinity Hall, Cambridge

Anne Harding, London First (to June 1997)

Judy Hargadon, NHS Executive, London Primary Care Support Force (to April 1997)

Peter Higgins, Anonymous Trust (to Dec. 1996)

Stephen Hill, Director, Capital Action

Rosemary Humphrays, City Parochial Foundation (to May 1996)

Frank Jackson, Finance Director, King's Fund

David Mathew, Director, New Academy of Business

Robert Maxwell, Chief Executive, King's Fund (to Dec. 1997)

John Plender, Financial Times Ltd

Professor Jennie Popay, Public Health Research & Resource Centre, University of Salford

Danny Silverstone, Director, London Boroughs Grants Unit

Linda Smith, Chairwoman, Lambeth, Southwark & Lewisham Health Authority

Diana Stent, NatWest Group

Perry Walker, New Economics Foundation

Sharon Welch, London First

Judie Yung, NHS Executive, North Thames Region (to Oct. 1997)

Operational Group

Directors: Pat Gordon and Diane Plamping

Many colleagues have contributed to the LHP initiative over nearly five years, some as members of the core group and others working mainly in local sites. They include Barbara Douglas, Kathryn Evans, Martin Fischer, John Harries, Iain Kitt, Sue Lloyd-Evelyn, Dave Martin, Jane Neubauer, Sharon Ombler Spain, Julian Pratt and Madeleine Rooke-Ley.

Annotated bibliography

Working whole systems

Brown E (1995) Well past 21 – a whole systems event based in general practice, *Primary Care Management*, 5, 10–11

Douglas B (1997) It's the elephant they never forget: a new approach to improving services for older people, *Working with older people*, July, 18–22

Gordon P (1998) Time is money for Watford carers, *Local Government Chronicle*, April 24, 15

Gordon P, Hanafin T (1998) Hands across the divide, *Health Management*, October, 20–1
From 'events' to 'this way of working'

Gordon P, Plamping D, Pratt J (1998) A sense of purpose, *Managing Care*, Dec, 6–7
A short account of the partnership typology

Harries J, Gordon P, Plamping D, Fischer M (1999) *Elephant problems and fixes that fail*, Whole Systems Thinking Working Paper Series (London, King's Fund)

Harries J, Gordon P, Plamping D, Fischer M. (1998) *Projectitis: spending lots of money and the trouble with project bidding*, Whole Systems Thinking Working Paper Series (London, King's Fund)

Jee M, Popay J, Everitt A, Eversley J (1999) *Developing Urban Primary Care: evaluating the London & Northern Health Partnership's 'Whole Systems Approach'* (Salford, Public Health Research & Resource Centre)

Moore W (1995) All hands to the slump – a user-friendly experiment in Croydon, *The Guardian*, 25 July

Newcastle Whole Systems (1997a) Common Strategy Document, *http://www.newcastle-city-council.gov.uk/wholesystems/gohome.htm*

Newcastle Whole Systems (1997b) *Going Home – making a common strategy work* Video and workbook (Newcastle, Barbara Douglas (0191 233 0200) or *wws@dial.pipex.com*)

Pascoe S, Pratt J (1998) Cold Remedies, *Health Service Journal*, December 10, 28–9

Whole system approach to winter beds pressure

Plamping D (1998) Change and resistance to change in the NHS, *British Medical Journal*, 317, 69–71

A first stab at a set of self-ordering principles that may underlie the way the NHS works

Plamping D, Gordon P, Pratt J (1998) *Action Zones and large numbers*, Whole Systems Thinking Working Paper Series (London, King's Fund)

Popay J, Williams G (1998) Partnership in health: beyond the rhetoric, *Journal of Epidemiology & Community Health*, 52, 410–11

Pratt J, Kitt I (1998) Going home from hospital – a new approach to developing strategy, *British Journal of Health Care Management*, 4, 391–5

Pratt J, Plamping D, Gordon P (1998) *Partnership: fit for purpose?*, Whole Systems Thinking Working Paper Series (London, King's Fund)

Pratt J, Plamping D, Ombler-Spain S, Harries J, Gordon P, Fischer M, Evans K (1998) *The NHS – Order for free? Proceedings from the Organisations as Complex Evolving Systems conference* (Warwick, BPRC)

Stewart M (1995) Health for all – the consumer's view, *Health for all news*, 32, 14–15

A lay participant's view of a Whole System Event

Wilkinson M (1999) *Creative Writing: its role in evaluation*, Whole Systems Thinking Working Paper Series (London, King's Fund)

Complex systems

Axelrod R (1984/1990) *The Evolution of Co-operation* (London, Penguin)

An application of game theory to social behaviour. It explores the conditions under which co-operation can emerge, including those where players remain 'selfish'.

Battram A (1998) *Navigating Complexity* (London, The Industrial Society)

An introduction to some of the theory and language of complexity, in particular how it relates to organisations.

Capra F (1996) *The Web of Life: a new synthesis of mind and matter* (London, Harper-Collins)

Provides a synthesis of ideas drawn from 'new science' and insights into their relevance to human development.

Goodwin B (1997) *How the Leopard Changed Its Spots: the evolution of complexity* (London, Phoenix)

An accessible explanation of how rich detail and diversity can be derived from simple rules.

Kauffman S (1995/1996) *At Home in the Universe: the search for the laws of complexity* (Harmondsworth, Penguin)

Provides a link between ideas in physics and maths and their expression in nature.

Kelly K (1994) *Out of Control: the new biology of machines* (London, Fourth Estate and USA, Addison Wesley)

Explores new ideas on the adaptability and autonomy of living organisms and their significance for human systems.

Maturana H, Varela F (1987/1992) *The Tree of Knowledge: the biological roots of human understanding* (Boston & London, Shambhala)

Describes the difference between organisation and structure in autopoetic systems.

Reynolds CW (1987) Flocks, herds and schools: a distributed behavioural model, *Computer Graphics*, 21, 25–34
see also *http://hml.com/cwr/boids.html*

Three simple rules tell animated 'birds' how to behave as a flock

Stewart I (1996) *Nature's Numbers: discovering order and pattern in the universe* (London, Phoenix)

An introduction to the mathematical underpinning of complex patterns in nature.

Tenner E (1996) *Why Things Bite Back: technology and the revenge effect* (London, Fourth Estate)

Unexpected consequences of intervening in complex systems

Methods – including Large Group Interventions

Bunker BB, Alban BT (1997) *Large Group Interventions – engaging the whole system for rapid change* (San Francisco, Jossey-Bass)

Provides an excellent introduction to Large Group Interventions and an overview of the best-known methods.

Cooperrider, Srivastva (1987) 'Appreciative inquiry into organisational life'. In: *Research in Organisational Change and Development*, Passmore and Woodman (eds) Vol 1 (Greenwich, JAI Press)

Cooperrider D (1997) *Appreciative Inquiry: a constructive approach to organisation development and change* (Case Western Reserve University)

Hammond SA (1996) *The thin book of appreciative inquiry*

A good place to start from to find out about appreciative inquiry – available from Anne Radford (AnneLondon@aol.com) who co-ordinates a network of UK practitioners of Appreciative Inquiry

Jacobs R (1994) *Real Time Strategic Change* (San Francisco, Berrett-Koehler)

Mindell A (1995) *Sitting in the Fire: large group transformation using conflict and diversity* (Portland, Lao Tse Press)

New Economics Foundation (1998) *Participation Works. 21 techniques of community participation for the 21st century* (London, NEF)

A source book for ideas about participative methods

Owen H (1992/97) *Open Space Technology: a user's guide* (San Francisco, Berrett-Koehler)

An accessible and enjoyable account of 'how to do it'. Romy Shovelton (romys@compuserv.com) co-ordinates a network of Open Space practitioners in the UK and organises training events.

Weisbord MR, Janoff S (1995) *Future Search: an action guide to finding common ground in organisations and communities* (San Francisco, Berrett-Koehler)

A clear account of the theory and practice of Future Search Conferences. More information at *http://www.searchnet.org*. UK contact is Perry Walker at the New Economics Foundation (Visions@neweconomics.org)

Organisations and organisational change

Checkland P, Scholes J (1990) Soft Systems Methodology in Action (Chichester, John Wiley)

Hamel G (1996) Strategy as revolution , *Harvard Business Review*, July–August, 69–82

Harrison A (1997) *The London Health Care System* (London, King's Fund)

Johnston, Russell, Laurence, Paul R (1988) Beyond vertical integration – the rise of the value-adding partnership, Harvard Business Review, July–August, 94–101

McMaster MD (1995/6) *The Intelligence Advantage: organising for Complexity* (Butterworth-Heinemann)

An approach to creating 'possibilities' for change within organisations based on the work of the Santa Fe Institute.

Morgan G (1986) *Images of organization* (Newbury Park, Sage Publications)

The use of metaphors in organisational life.

Normann R, Ramirez R (1994) *Designing interactive strategy* (Wiley)

An approach to organisational development for service industries based on the concept of co-production.

Penzias, Arno (1995) *Harmony* (Harper Business)

Rittel, Weber (1973) Dilemmas in a general theory of planning, *Policy Science* 4 155–69

This is the source of the terms 'tame and wicked problems' in planning and suggests appropriate responses to each.

Schon DA (1979) Public service organisations and the capacity for public learning, *Int Soc Sci J* XXXI 682–95

An analysis of why organisations fail to adapt.

Senge PM (1993) *The Fifth Discipline: the art and practice of the learning organization* (London, Century Business)

Based on experience gained from the MIT Centre for organisational learning, it applies ideas from system dynamics to organisational change.

Stacey RD (1996) *Strategic Management & Organisational Dynamics* (London, Pitman)

A broad overview of organisational development theories which describes their comparative strengths and limitations in practice.

Wheatley MJ (1992/4) *Leadership and the New Science: learning about organization from an orderly universe* (San Francisco, Berrett-Koehler)

Wheatley MJ, Kellner-Rogers M (1996) *A simpler way* (San Francisco, Berrett-Koehler)

A passionate plea for a new approach to understanding organisations and the way they work in the light of new ideas in science.

Others

de Shazer S (1998) *Clues: investigating solutions in brief therapy* (San Francisco, Norton)

The evidence supporting the effectiveness of identifying solutions without seeking to understand the causes of problems.

WHOLE SYSTEMS THINKING Working Papers

Projectitis
Spending lots of money and the trouble with project bidding

John Harries, Pat Gordon, Diane Plamping and Martin Fischer

Why does short-term investment in one-off projects seldom deliver the desired outcomes for organisational change? Why does the learning from demonstration projects seldom transfer to other places? This paper considers these conundrums and offers a different way of thinking about how to use development resources.

Price £5.00   ISBN 1 85717 211 6

Action Zones and Large Numbers
Why working with lots of people makes sense

Diane Plamping, Pat Gordon and Julian Pratt

Action zones will have to find ways of engaging the energy and commitment of large numbers of people. If they are to ëbreak the mouldí and deliver fundamental change, they will have to find genuinely new ways of working. This paper suggests a way of productively involving large numbers of people at every stage.

Price £5.00   ISBN 1 85717 226 4

Partnership: Fit for purpose?
Julian Pratt, Diane Plamping, Pat Gordon

Partnership between organisations is hard to achieve. There is often a mismatch between our aspirations for partnership and the frustration of our experience in practice. This paper offers a way of thinking about the purpose of partnership; partnership behaviours which fit different purposes; and partnership behaviours which can lead to sustainable change and are not dependant on injections of external resources.

Price £5.00   ISBN 1 85717 229 9

Creative Writing

Its role in evaluation

Margaret Wilkinson

Creative writing can provide a powerful tool in qualitative evaluation. The exercises and examples in this book are based on writing games, story telling and memory. They are affirming, problem-solving and democratising. Evaluation becomes something that everyone is asked to think about and take part in.

Price £5.00   ISBN 1 85717 228 0

Elephant Problems and Fixes that Fail

The story of a search for new approaches to inter-agency working

John Harries, Pat Gordon, Diane Plamping and Martin Fischer

This is the story of one group's struggle to develop a new approach to cross-boundary working. It starts from a growing dissatisfaction with change initiatives which fail to both learn the lessons of earlier investment and deliver desired outcomes. It recounts what shaped the way we did things, and why. It traces in particular the interplay of theory and practice and the search for practical ways of applying theories to the 'real world'.

Price £5.00   ISBN 1 85717 232 9

All titles in the Whole Systems Thinking series are available from:

King's Fund Bookshop
11–13 Cavendish Square
London W1M 0AN
Tel: 0171 307 2591